AMERICAN PHYSICAL THERAPY ASSOCIATION

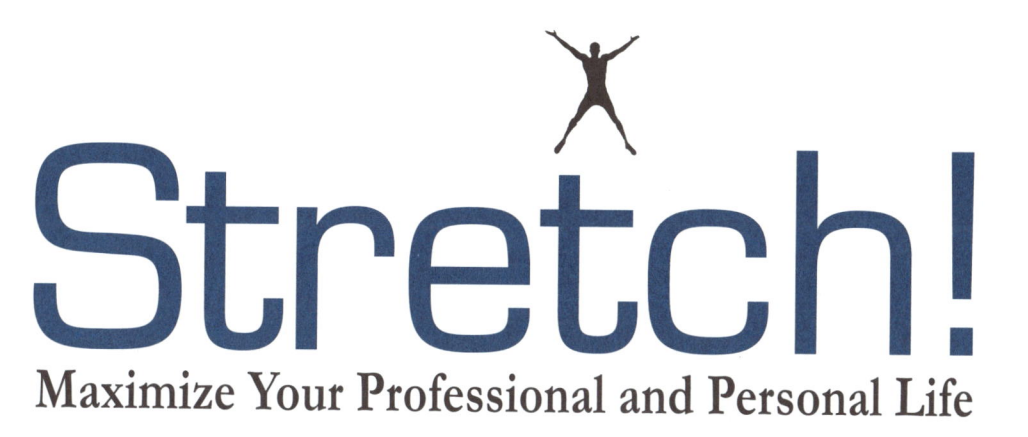

Stretch!
Maximize Your Professional and Personal Life

Brad Cooper, PT, MSPT, MBA, MTC, ATC
Editor: Eric Ries

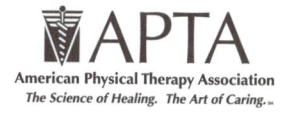

APTA
American Physical Therapy Association
The Science of Healing. The Art of Caring.

This compilation of articles originally was published in *PT—Magazine of Physical Therapy* ©2000, 2001, 2002, 2003, 2004, 2005, 2006.

ISBN 1-931369-29-1

©2006 by the American Physical Therapy Association.
All rights reserved.

For more information about this and other APTA publications, contact the merican Physical Therapy Association, 1111 North Fairfax Street, Alexandra, VA 22314-1488, 800/999-2782, ext 3395, www.apta.org.

[Order No. P-173]

Table of Contents

Introduction 1

Section 1
Back to Basics
Getting Down to Business 5
The 'Other' Net...................... 10
Service Matters!..................... 14
Review Your Performance Reviews! 18
Fitting Questions................... 23
Standing Out When Moving On 25

Section 2
Just Look at Yourself
Stuck in the Middle? 29
Escape! 35
Lessons Learned Along the Road................................. 40
Where's the Passion? 45
What's Your 'Fear Factor'? 49
A Resolution Revolution....... 52

Section 3
It's Your Attitude
Awakening the Wow!............. 55
The Success Cycle.................. 60
Beat Burnout!.......................... 65
How's That?............................. 70
The 'Other Side' of Goals...... 74
Look Beneath the Surface 77

Section 4
Sport as Life
Tendencies of an All-Star...... 81
'Tri'ed and True Tactics for Professional Success 87
When the Playing Field Changes 92
It's All Inside........................... 94
Subduing 'the Q'..................... 97
Going the Distance—and Then Some 99

Section 5
Personality Rules!
Appreciate the Differences! 103
So That's Why You Said That! 108
Get in Sync! 112

Section 6
Greet the Clock
It's About Time.................... 119
Don't Try Patients' Patience................................ 124
Are You Ready for a Revolution?.......................... 127
What's for Lunch? How About Innovation? 133
Up-to-the-Minute Advice... 135
Bringing It All Back Home 138

Section 7
Suggested Readings 141

Introduction

Seven years—33 columns. Wow! And now the excitement of a book, compiling the thoughts of one simple guy who's lived a life full of blessings over those years. Thoughts that hopefully helped a few folks along the way. As so often happens in life, that was never the plan. I remember sending a sample column to *PT Magazine* in 1999—it identified some of the potential pitfalls and possibilities for PTs or PTAs looking for their first or next professional move.

The editor liked it enough to continue. Readers responded to more columns. And the critics agreed they were worth a look (obviously thanks to great editing!): the American Society of Healthcare Publication Editors in 2001 bestowed its Gold Award on Career Coach as "Best Regular Column—Contributed." An accident? Maybe. Being in the right place at the right time? Probably. An enjoyable ride, thanks to people such as my editor Eric Ries [*PT Magazine's* associate editor, manuscripts] and so many other great folks at the American Physical Therapy Association? Absolutely.

But how often do such "accidents" happen to each and every one of us? Call it Chance. Call it Divine Guidance. Call it Luck. Each one of us—if our eyes are open to the opportunity—has things come into our lives every day that we never could have nor would have expected. That's not unique to me or anyone else. *The critical difference is what we do with those opportunities.* How will you seize the opportunity to better care for your next patient? Improve your relationships with colleagues? Set an example for a PT or PTA student or new graduate? Connect with your loved ones? Contribute to your Association and the profession? This compilation, if taken to heart, will help you to maximize your professional and personal pursuits, as well as your life.

It's up to you. You must make the choice. You must take that next step. *You* must choose to pursue excellence and leave mediocrity behind. *You*, and only you, are the one who has the opportunity to say "I want to sing my song—to be me—with all that I have."

One of my favorite songs of all time is *My Praise* by a little known group named Phillips, Craig and Dean. It talks about the fact that each one of us has something special to bring before our Maker. Not everyone can sing. Not everyone is a great athlete. Not everyone can lead effectively. But *everyone* brings some special gift to the table, and when we're utilizing that special gift, it is truly special indeed. Here's a little taste of the chorus:

Like an ocean breeze blowing on Your face

Like a summer sun with its warm embrace

Like a gentle rain plays a symphony

That's what I want my praise to be

Like a fragrant rose in the early spring

Like an eagle soars when it spreads it wings

Did you catch it? The ocean breeze is at its best when it's being what it was designed to be. The rose and the eagle have absolutely nothing in common. But when each are fully engaged in what they were created to be it's an incredible, majestic, amazing outcome.

So, what about you? What's your special gift? What were you created to be? To do? To add to your profession, your team, your community, your country, or beyond? You've seen it in people, haven't you? In business-speak, it's called "being fully engaged." In sports it's when someone is "in the zone." It appears almost effortless, yet the results are impressive.

One of the most enjoyable aspects of being a dad is watching our three kids find their gifts. Whether it's singing, performing a round-off back handspring, or making the world smile, they each have unique talents. And when they have an opportunity to really "be themselves"—to live out those talents and gifts—it's a beautiful thing to behold. But this is not unique to parenting. Whether it's watching an employee or student or child come into her own and excel in a specific area, or a runner glide across the track—seeing people discover who they are and put their gifts into practice—is, to me, my favorite of all types of art, an art that literally can change the life of both the individual and all those around him.

Thanks for picking up this book and making the decision to read it through. But please don't stop there. Put it through the ringer. Fold over the corners of pages that hit home. Underline and star the ideas that you can (will!) put into practice. Write notes in the back about how *you* can take your professional and personal life up another level by following some of the simple—and frankly timeless (they didn't start with me, I just put them into a format that might help get your attention)—suggestions noted inside.

And let me know how it's going (Results@wowspeak.com). I love to hear about your success stories. If the contents of this book result in just a handful of individuals making a little bit better use of what's been given to them, then it will have been worth the effort.

All the best to you as you turn another page.

Back to Basics

Getting Down to Business

PTs need to know the numbers to be successful in today's competitive job market.

In the novel *The Goal*[1] (definitely worth picking up!), the main character struggles to answer a consultant's question: "What is the goal of your organization?" The answer seems too obvious. The goal of the organization (in this case a manufacturing plant) is clearly to produce products, right? If that's the main objective, however, why worry about such things as limiting inventory and controlling operational expenses?

Why? Because a business's overriding goal is to make money—ethically and legally, of course. The novel's main character is a bit embarrassed that it takes him a while to reach this conclusion, but the consultant assures him he's not alone. Most people are slow to appreciate this simple fact. A business can have the best of motivations and do many things well, but if it doesn't make money it will have to close its doors. Even nonprofit organizations must closely monitor expenses in order to survive.

Now, make the jump to our profession. Physical therapists (PTs) are devoted to alleviating pain, preventing the onset and progression of limiting and disabling conditions, and promoting overall health and optimal quality of life. Our commitment to putting patients first is reflected in the profession's Code of Ethics and its Guide for Professional Conduct. (Both documents are available at www.apta.org.) The latter states in part that PTs are to be "guided at all times by concern for the physical, psychological, and socioeconomic welfare of those individuals entrusted to their care." Few if any PTs enter the profession strictly or even primarily for the money. But all PTs have a vested interest in, and an obligation to be at least somewhat knowledgeable about, the financial side of their facility or organization. The facility must pay its bills, just as you must in your personal life. Just as the bank that holds your mortgage isn't about to forgive your payments simply because you're a PT, it doesn't matter how outstanding the care you provide is if you can't afford the lease on your building. And if you can't pay the rent, your patients and clients may be forced to look elsewhere for the high-quality care you provide.

Too few PTs take the time to consider the various factors that influence their facility or organization's financial position, or what they can do to enhance that position. It all may seem complex and intimidating. A quick course in "Business 101," however, should remove much of the fear, mystery, and general confusion.

The Basics

> Every business has a "scorecard" that comes out each month. It's called a profit-and-loss statement.

Every business has a "scorecard" that comes out each month. It's called a profit-and-loss statement. It may look like a complicated document, but it's really not. In fact, in many ways it parallels your personal financial statements.

When you get your check at the end of a pay period, the amount you receive is less than the amount you "billed" your employer for your services. This is because before you even see the money, taxes have been removed. Similarly, your facility has something called contractual, or insurance, adjustments that reduce charges down to what the various insurance companies are actually going to pay your organization based on contracts. It parallels your own check stub.

After your taxes are removed from your paycheck, it's time to take out medical insurance and 401(k) or other retirement benefit "expenses." In the same way, a big expense category for your organization is salaries, which are substantial in any physical therapy organization because our primary "product" is time with a therapist.

If you're a homeowner, perhaps your biggest monthly bill is your mortgage. This is considered a "fixed" expense, because you can add family members without incurring additional mortgage costs—at least until your family has grown so large that you need a bigger house. Similarly, your facility very likely can add a significant number of additional patients before a new building is required. The important thing to remember about "fixed" expenses is that, on a per-visit basis, they actually go down as visits go up—just as the per-person cost of a mortgage goes down as the family grows.

So now you're left with such expenses as food, clothing, and entertainment—"variable" costs that change from month to month and are very dependent on the number of people under your roof. Back to the facility, and we're looking at expenses like delivery and supply costs that similarly vary from month to month based on the number of patient visits. Unlike fixed expenses, these variable costs go up as visits increase—just as a household's variable costs increase as the family grows—and are actually constant (at least in theory) on a per-visit basis.

So, it's really pretty simple. When you come down to it, running a business is in many ways similar to what you already do at home each month. And, as is the case at home, it's best if you can monitor your costs and do what you can to avoid financial trouble down the road.

Tracking Success

What are some key indicators that your life is going in the direction you want it to, and that you're reaching your personal goals? They may include the amount of time you spend with your spouse or children, the size of your nest egg, even your golf handicap or a 10K time you're determined to beat. However formally or informally, you keep track of these facts, figures and goals. Your organization also must identify and track indicators of success.

> I've often thought of having a T-shirt made that reads, "VISITS are life! Everything else is just details."

Have you seen the T-shirt that shouts in large print: "Baseball [or the wearer's favorite sport] is life! Everything else is just details"? I've often thought of having a T-shirt made that reads, "VISITS are life! Everything else is just details." That may be an overstatement, but in so many ways it's true! If you can keep your number of visits up, many of the other key expense factors, such as salary costs and fixed cost per visit, will take care of themselves. As the number of visits grows, your cost per visit actually drops sharply. The reason for this is the concept of marginal cost, which is not to be—but often is—confused with average cost.

Let's go back to the home example. If you have a family of three, you determine the average monthly cost per person by dividing all your costs by three. However, if a new child comes along, the marginal cost (the cost of the new addition) is much lower than the average cost per person up to that point (after getting past the original hospital bills, of course). The reason is that many of your expenses (house, car— even clothes, if hand-me-downs are an option) will remain constant with the new addition. Some expenses will increase (such as those for food, diapers, etc), but these constitute a much smaller figure than the average cost per person up to that point.

In the same way, the marginal cost at your clinic is the cost of the next patient to walk in the door. Think back to the profit-and-loss categories. Salary costs increase only if your staff is fully scheduled prior to the arrival of new patients; fixed costs are unlikely to change. That leaves just the remaining variable costs, which, in my experience, typically are just 15% to 20% of the average cost. So, the (marginal) cost of that next patient may be just 15% to 20% of what it cost to see all the patients up to that point!

Consider what you can do to help increase the number of visits, such as better marketing yourself and your facility to physicians, or getting entrepreneurial and developing a niche practice, as I discuss in "Tendencies of an All-Star." (See page 81.) When you're auditing the books, look for "lost" patients (those who were approved for six or eight visits but disappeared after two or three) to see why they stopped coming and what you can do about it.

But an increasing number of visits isn't the only indicator that your facility or organization is going in the right direction. Track these key factors as you seek to expand your facility's horizons:

- **Referrals (or new patients) per day.** This figure clearly is tied closely to visits, and can be used as a predictor of future visits. Consider using this number to gauge future coverage needs and maximize your use of time in the coming weeks.

- **Same-store growth.** This statistic compares monthly or year-to-date figures (either visits or referrals) to those for the same period in the previous year. It's a strong indicator of actual growth, as it takes seasonal trends into account. For example, your facility may be 30% busier in November than it is in October in terms of visits. If that's a seasonal trend in your area due to people having surgery and therapy before the health insurance deductible restarts, however, it's even more important to know how this November compares with last November—and not just to the number of visits the previous month. Same-store growth looks specifically at such seasonal trends.

- **Cancellation/no-show percentage.** As therapists, we can't simply put our time on the shelf for a client to pick up later. If you're in an outpatient arena and a significant percentage of patients are missing appointments, this has a substantial impact on the clinic's results financially (as well as the patient's progress clinically). See if you can get a baseline of other local clinics' and/or therapists' cancellation/no-show rates. If your rates are significantly (2% to 4%) above the norm, it's time to take a look at customer loyalty.

- *Cost per day/cost per visit.* In many settings (such as acute care), cost per day is a critical factor, because it's easily compared with revenue per visit to produce an average profit margin per visit. Incremental change up or down can have a significant impact on the facility's success.

A Little Knowledge Is a Great Thing

You can track the success of a majority of organizations and facilities by paying close attention to the factors listed in this column. Scrutinize them and you'll be way ahead of the curve.

If, for example, you're in the market for a PT position, you'll impress interviewers by having done some research in advance on which key statistics are most important to your prospective employer. (Intelligent questions along these lines will make you stand out in an interview!)

If you're already employed as a PT but don't tend to see much of the facility's "numbers," show your desire to learn and grow by asking about some of the figures discussed in this column. Volunteering to track a few of them regularly (a simple process once a spreadsheet has been set up) will instantly move you toward that all-star level I describe in "Tendencies of an All-Star."

And, if you're a supervisor who's hesitant to share such information with staff, please reconsider. Outside of salaries, which should always remain confidential, the more you share, the more members of your team will discover how each of them individually can help the facility meet its financial goals. True leadership demands a certain discontent with the status quo. If you cultivate a team of people who are well-acquainted with the numbers and their implications, they'll share your goal of moving beyond business as usual and on to greater success.

It's no longer the "good ol' days." Profit margins have thinned, and the therapist who thinks "good hands" are all that matter anymore is gravely mistaken. Spend some time getting down to business and you're certain to have a much more significant—and positive—impact on your organization and your own future.

Reference
1. Goldratt E. *The Goal.* Great Barrington, Mass: North River Press; 1984.

The 'Other' Net

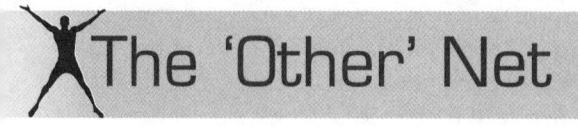

A solid network is a critical tool for all clinicians.

Pick up any magazine or newspaper, and you'd think the Internet is the answer to every problem facing the planet. And yes, it's a great—make that an *incredible*—tool. But there's another "net" that's even more important when it comes to developing a professional path: your net*work*.

Mom was right. It's not always *what* you know, but rather *who* you know that can have the biggest impact. Knowledge is important, but when a project needs to get done, is it the "smarts" or the connections that move the job along to completion the fastest? (Hint: Read "Standing Out When Moving On" on page 24, where I point out that somewhere in the neighborhood of 80% of all job offers are a result of knowing the right person, not the right stuff.) Whether you're seeking a job, considering the need for a professional change, or want to be prepared "just in case," you need to hone your networking skills.

What's a network? Very simply, it's a compilation of all of the people you know and all of the people *they* know (if you know that they know them, of course). Statistics indicate that most people have at least 250 contacts.[1] Picture multiplying your skills, knowledge, and talent by that figure a few times (and yes, feel free to use a calculator), and the impact is obvious. That's the key to a network. It combines everyone's skills, talents, and knowledge into a world-changing machine. And please realize that it involves *two-way* communication and sharing of abilities. If you're looking to build a network just to "get," then you're barking up the wrong redwood.

Getting Started

Thomas Edison once said, "Everything comes to him who *hustles* while he waits." (No, not "hustling" others, but getting yourself moving.) That's really what networking is all about. Growing a network doesn't necessarily mean doing different things. Instead, it simply means doing the same things differently.

For example, my family regularly attends a local church. However, for years, we would come in, sit down, listen, and leave after the service. The result was nourishment for the soul, but no impact on the network.

Then, a few years ago, I discovered the value of networking. While I didn't completely give up my introvert tendencies, I began to make an effort to meet at least one person before the service and another afterward. Writing the names down helped my memory in ensuing weeks. Suddenly, the people I'd seen several times but whose names I couldn't ever remember (did I ever even know them?) were folks I could greet by name and get to know better over time. A few have even made it into my Rolodex™ (but we'll get to that later). Has my purpose in attending church changed? Of course not! But as long as I'm there, why not do more than fill up a seat?

In the same way, when you attend a seminar or any other event, you don't need to transform into some sort of artificial shmoozer. But, as long as you're there anyway, you should make good use of the time by making some contacts. The point is that it took *no* additional time to grow my network in this setting, just a purposeful move out of my comfort zone.

And that's just one example. The same application can be made to any setting: APTA functions, sporting events, the line at the movies, the pool, the golf course, the elevator, on an airplane—anywhere! It just takes practice, practice, *practice*.

The Next Step

Okay, so you can handle meeting a few extra people at places you already frequent, and you're ready to dive head-first into networking. Where do you start? There probably are no better training wheels for networking than Chamber of Commerce meetings. Every town has them, and practicing your new-found networking skills in this setting is simple, educational, and free of intimidation.

Networking at a Chamber meeting is like discussing football at a Super Bowl party. Even if you have little idea of what to say, people will ask you about your business and for your card. After a few lessons in this setting, you'll be ready to give it a try anywhere.

Like anything, preparation is key. Before arriving at the meeting, come up with a curiosity statement for your name tag that will get the ball rolling. As a career coach, I might write "Get a Job!" or "Move Ahead!" on my name tag, begging the question about what I have to offer. In a meeting I attended last month, a gentleman wrote "Golf Lessons" in big print on his name tag (his company combined golf lessons with networking high-level clients). He was busy all night explaining what he did to people for whom the word "golf" jumped off his chest.

Another item to prepare in advance is your own "30-second commercial" (with pizzazz) about what you have to offer. After your "commercial," you can ask the person if he or she has an interest in learning more about what you do. If not, the two of you can keep talking, or you can both move on without having spent too much time privately thinking "Who cares?"

However, before you even consider jumping into your "commercial," you need to remember the most important aspect of networking: *listening*. It's not new information that people like talking about themselves. If you learn to ask good questions and then really listen, networking will be a snap.

Once you've practiced a little at Chamber meetings, you're ready for application of your new skills elsewhere. The basics are the same. Be prepared, be genuine, and listen well. If you apply these, you'll be successful growing your network in any setting.

And don't miss an opportunity because you're looking for the perfect opener. Simple questions or statements like "How did you get involved with this organization?" or "I didn't realize there'd be this many people here" will get the ball rolling.[1] Remember, despite outward appearances, most people are just as timid as you are. Some of them have just practiced a little more.

Don't Stop There

Meeting people is just the beginning. The critical step is what comes next: the recording. If you don't already have a Rolodex,™ Blackberry, or some other type of recording method, put this article down right now and get one. It can be paper or electronic—the form doesn't matter, but the follow-through does.

Begin by going beyond the typical information (name and phone number). Use the entire card (the reason I like the *big* cards or an electronic system) to add other information you gather, such as spouse's name, kids' ages, clinical expertise, hobbies, and other information that will make your next meeting less like a cold call and more like renewing a friendship.

Once you get the process started, it's time to manage it. At least once a month (if not more), go through and update your new tool with your contacts' major job or personal changes, especially a move. Make plans to renew relationships with people you haven't contacted recently, with a lunch or even just a simple note. And most of all, nurture your "Rolodex™ community."[2] Harvey MacKay[3] emphasizes this, saying, "If there is any single rule to follow…it's *not* 'How can I get the other person to do something for me?'… it's 'How can I do something for the other person?'" As a therapist, an easy way to nurture a relationship with other clinicians might be something as simple as sending a colleague an article related to his or her specialty or special interest, along with a brief note.

Tom Peters, in his outstanding book *The Brand You 50*,[2] makes it very clear that *you are your Rolodex* (his description, but I like it!). Listen to Tom: "I could lose my luggage. Pain. No big deal. I could lose my wallet. Big Pain. No big deal. I could lose this manuscript. Huge Pain. Big Deal. Survivable. But if I lost my

Rolodex...I might consider hari-kari. Seriously. (Almost)." A well-managed Rolodex is a powerful thing.

And Finally...

Before you run out the door to your next networking opportunity, consider Gary Harvey's "Five Networking Sins."[4] They'll come in handy for any outside event, from a PT seminar to an Association meeting to your child's soccer game:

- Spending too much time with your friends at an event,
- Having no goal or objective (lack of preparation),
- Making no agreement with people you meet about future contact,
- "Telling" rather than "listening," and
- Not following up.

Keep these in mind the next time (*today*!) you have an opportunity to connect with someone new. Effective networking is not reserved for the naturally extroverted, but for the properly prepared. MacKay's statement to "network as if your life depended on it, because it does" isn't all that far off. With a little preparation, practice, and patience, you'll soon have a valuable network in place that will have an even bigger impact on your future than that "other" net!

References
1. Fisher D, Vilas S. *Power Networking*. Austin, Texas: MountainHarbour Publications; 1991.
2. Peters T. *The Brand You 50*. New York, NY: Random House; 1999.
3. MacKay H. *Dig Your Well Before You're Thirsty*. New York, NY: Doubleday; 1997.
4. Harvey G. Networking Smart. Presented at: Denver Chamber of Commerce meeting; January 27, 2000; Denver, Colorado.

Service Matters!

Here are common-sense tips for uncommon service to all your customers.

"Wow, what incredible service!" When was the last time those words passed through your lips on your way out the door of a business? It's been a while, hasn't it? We like to believe good customer service is simply good common sense. It may be, but that certainly doesn't make it common.

Does customer service really make a difference in today's fast-paced health care environment? You'd better believe it does! In fact, you may be surprised to know that Microsoft Chairman Bill Gates, whose entire organization is built on and around technology, states in his book, *Business @ the Speed of Light: Succeeding in the Digital Economy*[1] that nothing is more important to any organization than good old customer service. If it's that important to a "hands off" company like his, shouldn't it be considerably more important to us, as health care providers who work one-on-one with patients at critical times in their lives?

Just as physical posturing has a tremendous impact on the effective movement of the body, your "mental posturing" has an incredible effect on how you work with those around you.

The Customer

Who is your customer, anyway? Patients immediately come to mind, of course, and maybe physicians. But what about case managers? Coworkers? Your supervisor? How about patients' families?

The simple act of identifying your customer is a good start on the road to providing great customer service. Something as simple as changing your mindset to consider someone such as a coworker or case manager a "customer" can change your outlook on and your actions toward that person. And, just as physical posturing has a tremendous impact on the effective movement of your body, your "mental posturing" has an incredible effect on how you work with those around you.

For example, think back to the toughest patient you've seen in the past couple of weeks. If you were to walk by the front door and see her coming from her car toward your facility, what would you tell yourself to position your mental posturing? Would you say, "Oh, no—here comes Mrs. Jones again. I can't stand working with that woman." Or, would you say, instead, "There's Mrs. Jones. She had a rough day the other day. I bet this injury is really affecting her ability to do the things she enjoys. I think I'll see if I can get her to walk out with a smile today."

Similarly, when it comes to your coworkers, what types of questions or comments typically come out of your mouth when you walk in the door in the morning? The first thing you say can set the tone for the entire day. If you come in with a proverbial chip on your shoulder, wishing you were somewhere else, it shows. (And your coworkers will probably wish you were somewhere else, too!)

Last year, I gave a brief talk on the importance of mental posturing to a group of employees and later that day visited their clinic. When I walked in the door, the receptionist enthusiastically asked, "Brad, are you having a *great* day?" Then, as I walked around the corner, one of the physical therapists (PTs) poked his head out of the room and said, "Isn't it an awesome day? How's it going?" While I was still absorbing this onslaught of positive energy, a third person greeted me with, "Hi! What a *fantastic* day!"

Was this team purposely taking it to the extreme, for my benefit? Sure. But I'll tell you what—after a couple of days of displaying such enthusiasm, it started (at a slightly lower level of intensity) to become a habit. When I walk into that clinic now, I can't help but smile, expecting to enjoy my time with some great people who keep the positive energy flowing. It really does make a difference!

Whatever type of customer you're serving, your mental posturing affects your actions. Too often, we just go with our natural, reflexive response to those around us, which may not be particularly positive or customer service oriented. Instead, we should try thinking about the impression we're leaving and the example we're setting.

Two Ears, One Mouth

It's been said that God knew what he was doing when he gave us two ears and one mouth. All of us should take the hint and listen at least twice as much as we talk. Michael Leboeuf shares the following "IOU" memory trick in his audiotape, *How to Win Customers and Keep Them for Life*:[2]

- *I* is to remind you that maintaining *eye* contact is extremely important.
- *O* is to remind you to let the speaker know you're listening by responding with an occasional "*oh*," "okay," "uh-huh," or "right" while he or she is talking.
- *U* is to remind you that it's good to show you've been listening by saying things like, "So, what *you* see as being the solution here is … ."

Section 1 — Back to Basics   **15**

Whatever method you use to help you focus on listening, it's critical to outstanding customer service. Still not convinced? Try this: The next time you meet someone new, forget trying to impress him with your vast knowledge and experience. Just listen to what he has to say, encourage him to tell you more, and close the encounter by praising him in some way. He'll have dominated the conversation, but he'll walk away thinking you're one of the nicest people he's ever met!

The Service

Simply stated, customers want two things: good feelings and solutions to problems. PTs and physical therapist assistants (PTAs) have a unique opportunity to meet both of these needs. But are you meeting them consistently? The better you can do so, the more successful you'll be. Great ability in the clinic goes a long way, but if you lack "bedside manner," your overall effectiveness in meeting your patients' needs will be greatly limited. The PT or PTA who can combine exceptional technical ability with compassionate patient care is going to have a lot of happy customers.

Jeffrey Gitomer lays it on the table in the title of his book, *Customer Service Is Worthless, Customer Loyalty Is Priceless*.[3] For so long, we've been attempting to "satisfy" customers. But what we've failed to realize is that simple "satisfaction" doesn't cut it. A "satisfied" customer walks out the door saying, "Well, that was okay; nothing went particularly wrong." But a loyal customer is wowed and proceeds to tell everyone about the virtues of your organization. Will a loyal customer return if he or she needs further physical therapy? You bet! By comparison, the "satisfied" customer may return to you only if you're the most convenient option.

Ten Commandments

In our profession, many of our clients are in pain. Many, too, are worried about the potential effects of their injury or dysfunction on their careers and their finances. As a result, you may face clients who are less congenial than the average customer. When you do, keep these "Ten Commandments" in mind:

I. *Don't* let yourself be drawn into acting defensive. It never helps your cause to assert that you're "right" and suggest that the client may be "wrong." Remind yourself of the client's pain and focus on "taking care" instead of "taking offense."

II. *Don't* interrupt, even if you've heard it all "a million times" from other clients. If the patient starts repeating himself, try summarizing what he said (the "U" in the IOU example). This shows him that he's made his point, and then hopefully you won't have to listen to his point repeatedly.

III. *Don't* ever say, "I know how you feel." You don't! Instead, try saying something like, "I can see that you're upset by this whole situation, and I think I might feel the same way if I were in your situation."

IV. *Do* address the client's emotional needs first. As I noted earlier, customers want two things—good feelings and solutions to problems (and usually solutions to problems provide good feelings, so maybe it's really all one thing). Clients need to feel that you care about them just as much as they need your logical, problem-solving side.

V. *Do* stand up when the client approaches you—this simple body language reinforces that you're serious about focusing on his or her problem.

VI. *Do* try to make the client feel more comfortable with you by emulating him in subtle ways. If he's sitting down, for example, sit next to him. If he's leaning back, do the same. If he's looking you in the eye, meet his gaze. People tend to relate better to those with whom they feel some commonality, even if it's on a subconscious level.

VII. *Do* ask, "So that we can resolve the situation that's upsetting you, do you mind if I ask you a few questions?" This tells the client at the outset that you want to help, and that you want to do so now. By focusing the discussion in this way, you'll not only convey your concern, but you'll also get at the root of the problem (and hopefully its solution) that much more quickly.

VIII. *Do* explain to the upset client that you're going to document all the information he's telling you for follow-up, and then begin writing. This shows him that he's being taken seriously and is likely to calm him down.

IX. *Do* repeat some of the information back as you're taking notes, and offer a couple of possible solutions from which the client can choose, allowing her to feel more in control of the situation. For example, if the client is upset that she can "never" get an appointment at the end of the day, explain that while you understand her frustration, many clients seek late afternoon appointments. Offer to schedule her further in advance, or to contact a nearby clinic that has late afternoon slots available. You also might offer her a Saturday appointment if that's a viable option.

X. *Do* try to take at least some action immediately. For example, if the client has a concern about billing, consider following up on it with your billing office right away and leaving the client a voicemail message within the hour relating what you've done and when the matter is likely to be resolved—or at least what the next step will be.

The Payoff

The results you can gain by addressing a problem effectively are incredible. According to Leboeuf, fully 70% of initially dissatisfied customers will work with you again if you solve the problem. Ninety-five percent will work with you again if you solve it on the spot. If they remain dissatisfied when they complete their business with you, however, the chances are they won't come back!

One final note. We've probably all experienced how a top-notch "first impression team member" (receptionist, in some circles) can radically affect a patient's view of the overall level of care. That first impression often truly affects how the client views the whole organization. Keep in mind that providing great customer service requires an entire team—not just the PT—and that all clinic personnel would do well to heed the advice in this column.

If you establish "service beyond a smile" as a priority throughout the organization, the results will be impressive. From the client's initial phone call to treatment and through the billing process, service matters!

References
1. Gates B. *Business @ the Speed of Thought: Succeeding in the Digital Age.* New York, NY: Warner Books; 2000.
2. Leboeuf M. *How to Win Customers and Keep Them for Life* [audiotape]. New York, NY: Simon and Schuster; 1997.
3. Gitomer J. *Customer Satisfaction Is Worthless, Customer Loyalty Is Priceless.* Austin, Texas: Bard Press; 1998.

Review Your Performance Reviews!

Managers, follow these steps to transform performance reviews from empty exercises into meaningful, productive exchanges.

Most organizations *throw away* many hours of productivity two or more times a year while they go through the performance-review process with their employees. No, the words "throw away" aren't an exaggeration. In their current format, most performance reviews are, for all practical purposes, almost a complete waste of time—outside of the fact that they force supervisors to actually sit down with the employee and talk, something that might not happen otherwise.

If you think I'm guilty of overstatement, think back to the most-recent performance review you conducted. No, wait—let me see how close I can come to guessing what happened. You sat down with the employee for the first time in more than a month and went through a form that vaguely overlapped what the employee really does in his or her position. Somewhere within the process there was a list of strengths and weaknesses (being an enlightened manager, you likely referred to the latter as "areas for growth"). Then, at the end of review, you gave the employee some goals to pursue, and probably some steps by which to pursue those goals.

Unfortunately, the "areas for growth" listed for the employee undoubtedly were more a reflection of your own strengths than the employee's true growth needs. If you don't believe me, pull out a copy of that most-recent performance review and take a close look at it. Are you strong in the areas of marketing, manual therapy skills, and interpersonal communication? Then most likely—unless you hired the employee specifically because he or she was exactly like you—you listed those skills under the employee's areas for growth. And the self-improvement steps outlined along with the goals? Most likely they're perfect for a carbon copy of you. But how well do they actually work for the employee?

Of course, because the performance review often is tied to an immediate or potential raise, the employee probably simply nodded, took his or her medicine, and moved on. It's doubtful, however, that this investment of time did much of anything to illuminate the employee's weaknesses and encourage the development of his or her strengths.

My objective in writing these recommendations isn't to come down hard on managers. Managing is a tough job—something yours truly has learned as much through making mistakes as by any other means. On the other hand, though, maybe coming down on managers should be my objective. Those of us who manage employees carry an immense responsibility, after all. If all managers truly understand that responsibility and take it seriously, they'll learn how important the performance review process really is to everyone—by giving managers and employees alike an opportunity to shine in their respective roles.

Five Steps

What's the best way to fashion a performance review that truly will help the individual employee (and your team) attain a higher level of excellence, whether the employee is a clinician or a first-impression team member (receptionist)? Are you ready to revive and reinvigorate your facility by revamping your performance reviews—the cornerstone of the employer-employee relationship? If so, tighten your seatbelt and consider the following:

1. **Break the mirror!** A poll Marcus Buckingham cites in his book, *Now, Discover Your Strengths*,[1] showed that only 20% of people surveyed marked "strongly agree" in response to the statement, "You have a chance every day to do what you do well." In essence, that means only 20% get to be themselves each day! The other 80% are trying to be someone else—their supervisor, their parent, their professor, etc. How effective is that likely to be? (Hint: Have you ever seen a fish climb a tree? You get the idea.)

   Allow (force!) your team members to be themselves—not a mirror image of you! Most people feel they rarely get the chance, in any given work day, to fully use their strengths and operate in their own style. Managers, ask yourselves: What are you doing to make certain this isn't true of your team?

   Do team members have an opportunity to pursue tasks in ways that are completely different from the established norm, as long as the outcome is consistent with the expected results? Or is there an unwritten policy that it's "my way or the highway"? If so, make it clear during the review process that the "highway" has just been resurfaced and that optional routes are now available—and even encouraged.

2. **Break another mirror!** So you're tuned into the fact that not every employee goes about things the same way you do. What do you know about their attitudes toward professional advancement and taking on additional responsibilities? Are you aware that their plans for the future might be different from what you envision for them? To bring this out, draw a line on a piece of paper that climbs gradually, then starts to level off. Ask the employee where he thinks he is right now on that line. Does he see himself as being on the upward arc (in an advancement phase)? Starting to plateau? On a plateau?

   Don't stop there, however. The next, critical step is to ask the employee where he or she would *like* to be. If she's on a plateau, would she like to embark on a curve upward? Or maybe he'd like to slow down and plateau a little. Or possibly she's on the plateau and likes it there. The important thing to understand is that although you may be on a fast track to the top, constantly taking on new challenges, that doesn't mean that's everyone's goal.

   Once you've opened up this subject, a discussion of "what can we do together to make this happen" will naturally ensue.

3. ***Shred to get ahead!*** Put the current review through the shredder and start over! Take a look at the most-recent reviews you completed on two completely different people. How similar do the reviews appear to be, in terms of goals and the ways they were to be pursued? If you helped to design a strategy for pursuing the goals, it's extremely likely the strategy mimicked your style rather than reflecting the strategic style of the person charged with meeting the goals.

   For example, because you are skillful at gaining patient/client referrals by socializing with physicians in informal settings, your tendency might be to encourage an employee to help meet the clinic's growth goals by having lunch with two different physicians each week. Instead of projecting your own strategy onto the employee, however, seek his or her ideas on how to address the goal. The employee might present a strategy that is more in sync with his or her natural style and thus may promise better results than would simply mimicking your method.

   Work with the employee on goal-achievement strategies, zeroing in on the best way for that person to accomplish the goals. The result will be a greatly enhanced long-term outcome in terms of employee happiness and productivity, which is what you were looking for anyway, right?

4. ***Haste exacerbates the waste!*** Another unfortunate performance-review tradition in most workplaces is to schedule all of them—whether you have a staff of three or 50—for the same month or even the same week. Then, because you're unable to wave your magic wand and limit all of your "regular" work during this period, you must squeeze in all the performance reviews on top of your regular patient-care schedule and other tasks. The result? Despite your best intentions, the performance reviews become something you just need to "get done." (Translation: The quality and value of the evaluations tend to suffer.)

   What was the reason for this mad rush, again? Oh yeah, tradition. "We did it that way last year, and the year before that." Well, so what? Don't shortchange your staff, your facility, and yourself by dashing through the review process just for tradition's sake. Instead, change the tradition!

   Granted, employee reviews often help determine raises, so that may force some grouping of reviews within a general time period. With a little planning, however, you still can space them out better than clumping them all into the same week or 10 days. Also, why not begin the process well in advance—even if it's just completing some of the basics, such as starting the process of rating the employee in such categories as attitude, work ethic, and so on? That way, you can invest additional time in the critical strategy portion of the review as the time draws near.

5. **Get outta there!** Rather than conducting the review in your office, consider scooting out for a walk, a cup of coffee, or breakfast. A change of surroundings makes the time more special in the eyes of the employee, gets you way from phone calls and other interruptions, and allows you to focus completely on this specific—and important—team member. Just as couples need to get out for an occasional "date night" in the midst of their busy lives in order to keep the fire burning, a few moments of focused time with each of your team members is good for the soul—both yours and theirs.

Lead the Revival!

It should come as no surprise that when the Center for Creative Leadership conducted a 3-year study of the differences between top leaders and those who are marginally effective, a single difference emerged: top leaders demonstrate through their words and actions that they really care about their employees.[2] If you'll make the time to create a truly meaningful performance review, you'll be well on the way to demonstrating to your employees that you truly care about them.

So, what's it going to be? The same ol' same ol', or reviews that fuel a biannual revival within your team? If you're not ready to go the new route, save yourself some time and simply ask your staff to photocopy last year's performance-review form and give it a quick once-over. But if you're up for a performance review that will make a difference, remember: The revival starts with one person—you!

References
1. Buckingham M, Clifton DO. *Now, Discover Your Strengths*. New York, NY: Free Press; 2001.
2. Cooper RK. *The Other 90%: How to Unlock Your Vast Untapped Potential for Leadership and Life*. New York, NY: Crown Publishing; 2001.

Fitting Questions

Here are some keys to exploring your professional options in a conducive job market.

Have you noticed? You're a hot commodity again! That's not to imply that physical therapists (PTs) haven't been in demand over the last decade or so—the need for talented, hard-working PTs always has been high. But now we're seeing supply-and-demand levels reminiscent of the late 1980s and early 1990s.

An upswing in demand is an ideal time to evaluate your professional future. Your options may be more numerous than they have been in years. At the same time, however, it's important to realize the cyclical nature of employment trends. A job market that's sizzling with opportunity now may cool down considerably in a few years.

As you weigh your professional options—whether you're eyeing your next job or your first one—the key question is personal fit. The following are some key considerations.

Practice setting. What will it be? Acute care? Orthopedics? Pediatrics? Neurology? The conventional answer is that you should start in a position that allows you to work in various settings. But I say "baloney!" That's what clinical affiliations are for—they're outlets for test-driving areas of personal interest and expertise. Don't get me wrong—you might enjoy a diverse schedule that encompasses several settings. But, in choosing a position, don't go for diversity of settings just because you've always heard "that's the best way to start." Rather, ask yourself where you want to be in 5, 10, or 15 years. If you feel strongly that acute care, say, is the setting for you, don't wait to get started!

Type of facility. Once you're clear about your area of interest and expertise, it's time to decide what type of facility best fits you. Will you be working in a hospital or a free-standing facility, for example? The difference can be greater than you might imagine. Even if you're doing essentially the same things at both places, where you physically work can play a big role in determining the office culture, future employment opportunities, and more.

Tour some facilities. Ask questions about expectations of staff, work schedules, and opportunities for professional growth. Find out whether you'll have a chance to make a personal impact on the way the facility is run, should you see room for improvement or have innovative ideas. Ask PTs to walk you through their typical day—inasmuch as any day is "typical"—and seek insights into what challenges and energizes them.

Also, as you tour various job sites, keep in mind that, generally speaking, the line between for-profit and not-for-profit operations has blurred significantly over the years. Non-profit organizations have realized that they, too, must carefully monitor expenses and productivity if they are to survive in today's marketplace.

Leadership. Is there any? Who's in charge? What motivates him or her? Is the motivational standard closer to the "principle-centered leadership" of Stephen Covey's Seven Habits of Highly Effective People or to "seagull leadership"—you know, fly in, make a bunch of noise, leave behind a big mess, and then disappear? How long has the leader been there? How long has the team been together? What's the turnover level among those who report to that leader? What's the leader's communication style?

Also, should you be interested in pursuing a leadership role, what's the chain-of-command mechanism for doing that? What types of mentoring opportunities are available to potential leaders?

Don't make the mistake of failing to take into account the leadership qualities of your potential boss. Often, people don't quit their job so much as they quit their supervisor. I cannot stress enough the importance of identifying a supervisor who will support and nurture you and the facility in ways that you personally respect.

Benefits. Obvious—and important—questions to ask include, "What's the salary?" "How many vacation days will I receive?" And "Do you offer a 401(k)?" But don't forget to inquire about benefits that may be equally important in the big picture.

For example, if you are a hard-working, organized, and driven individual, perhaps you should be more concerned about whether the organization offers performance bonuses than about base salary. With few exceptions, salaries will fall within the same general range for the same type of job in the same region of the country. A $2,000 difference in annual starting wage between two similar jobs may seem like a lot to a new graduate, but keep in mind that that's not much per paycheck, after taxes. By comparison, a performance-driven bonus program easily could net conscientious workers much more than $2,000 in a year's time. Also, does the organization offer loan forgiveness? That's another huge potential benefit, depending on your circumstances.

Too many PTs rush through the interviewing process with little more than a cursory look at critical factors that can mean the difference between a long, successful stay and a brief, miserable stop along a bumpy professional road. There's no better time to explore your options than while the demand for PTs is high. Doing your homework not only will impress potential employees with your approach, but it also will better ensure long-term success in your next—or first—professional position.

Standing Out When Moving On

There are opportunities for professional advancement in today's employment market. How do you take advantage of them?

Not so very long ago, a physical therapist (PT) could practically scribble down his or her credentials, fax them out, and receive multiple job offers. Things have changed. If you want to practice in today's marketplace, you've got to be good—and I don't just mean a good PT.

Although national publications continue to rate careers in the field of physical therapy at the top of their lists in terms of future growth, finding a position is not an easy process. But, if you can put the same effort and investment into the job search that you put into your degree, you will find that there are opportunities available. How do you take advantage of these opportunities? Start at the beginning.

Networking

The beginning—that must mean résumés, right? Wrong. Step one is networking. When it comes to capturing a job, that old advice, "It's not what you know, but who you know that counts," certainly holds true.

Harvey MacKay, author of *Dig Your Well Before You're Thirsty*,[1] is the king of networking. Get the book, or at least ponder the title. Do you go out to dig your well when you start to feel a little thirsty? Of course not—it's too late by then. But far too often, we ignore the importance of building a network until the day we get that diploma or receive notice that our position has been eliminated. If you consider that more than 80% of filled positions probably are a result of knowing the right person[2] (not a result of the perfect résumé) it's clear that networking before you need it is worth the effort!

Whether or not you're currently in the job market, start expanding that Rolodex. At continuing education courses, state or national meetings, church, your kid's soccer tournament, or a gardening show, take notes about folks you meet and then transfer the information into a single location (electronic or card-based recording system). You say you don't have the time? You're already there—you're already having the conversation. The extra 1% of effort it takes later to transfer it into your permanent records is certain to pay off down the road.

One other note about networking: Many people unfortunately view a network as a way to "get" things, using social contacts to later take advantage of others. An effective network must go both ways. So, as you review your contact list occasionally, consider if there are any ways in which you can assist those in your network. Then, if you ever do need a helping hand, the recipient likely will be more than happy to return the favor. If you never need to ask for help, all the better.

The Cover Letter

Once your network is in place, the next step is researching and putting together a cover letter. Cover letters come in all shapes and sizes. As a career coach to PTs, I've seen about all types. There's no such thing as a perfect cover letter, but there certainly are many things that can be red flags to the person reviewing your letter, sending yours into the round file without a second look. Some of the most common include:

- *"To whom it may concern"* (or something similar) as a salutation. You might as well start off your letter saying, "I didn't want to take the time to find out to whom this letter should be sent. This job wasn't important enough to invest 3 minutes in making a phone call" (especially if you're searching from the same calling area!).

- *Spelling errors* (and you'd be surprised how many cover letters and résumés have these). Remember, "spell-check" won't catch everything, nor will you. Have someone else review your letter for you. Read it backward yourself for errors to avoid skimming through specific sections.

- *No indication as to what you'll add to the organization.* In *The Circle of Innovation*,[3] Tom Peters writes of the importance of every person being able to demonstrate why he or she makes the organization better than it would be without him or her. This means going beyond the basic credentials and highlighting the talents (for example, leadership or entrepreneurialism) and skills (for example, clinical specialization or advanced manual skills) that make you an outstanding candidate. This is especially true in our field, and even more so when you're seeking to be added to a team.

The Résumé

Your network is strong (or at least growing), you've got a solid cover letter in place, and now it's time to put together that résumé. Again, you'd be amazed at some of the samples I've seen. If you're responding to an advertisement, you may be one of 50 or more respondents. The recipient is likely looking for one of two things—outstanding characteristics that fit perfectly into the organization or reasons to screen people out. It's unlikely that, of the 50, more than 7 or 8 respondents will receive phone interviews, and 2 to 4 will get as far as live interviews. Your goal in this stage is either to show why you're the perfect fit (if you know you are), or at least to keep from being eliminated as a result of typos or inconsistencies. A few tips to consider:

- *Lead with your strength.* If your experience is outstanding, make sure it's toward the top of your résumé, leaving education for the middle or end (and vice-versa if your advanced degrees/credentials are your strength).

- *Keep the "core" of the résumé to one page* (although an attachment of one or more pages for continuing education or publications is very appropriate in our profession). Again, it's unlikely anyone's going to read more than the first page when screening through a stack of résumés. Don't take a chance that the important stuff never got read because it was on page 2!

- *Start off with a strong, well-stated profile or objective,* but make certain it fits the organization that will be receiving the résumé!

- *Make sure the appearance of the résumé is sharp.* It's part of that all-important first impression.

The Interview

You made the first cut! The invitation came for the interview. What now? Focus on the key word: preparation.

- *Do your research.* When you walk in the door, you should know more about that company (and maybe even the interviewer) than the average employee. This will always make you stand out as a candidate.

- *Arrive on time.* Practice driving to the interview location in traffic prior to the interview date to ensure you arrive early for the interview. There are plenty of excuses for being late, but an interviewer may assume that if a person can't be on time when on his or her best behavior, it's certain to be a problem later. Being late to an interview often is an automatic disqualifier for the job.

- *Know your strengths* and how to converse about them naturally. Nobody wants a conceited employee. But you'll never even get a chance if you are unable to express why you're the best fit for the position. I encourage therapists to review potential questions that may be asked but not to memorize answers, which only makes you appear robotic in your response.

- *Look sharp, and practice introductions.* It's been shown that first impressions are determined in the first 7 seconds and that decisions about candidates are often made within the first 5 minutes of the interview.[4]

If you start off poorly, a recovery may not be possible in time to save your opportunity.

- ***Don't assume anything*** about how well or how poorly the interview is proceeding. You have no idea how the other candidates did. I remember speaking with one woman about her interview. She told me how poorly she had performed. When I spoke later with the interviewer, he waxed eloquent about how she'd had an outstanding interview, resulting in her being one of the top candidates!

The process of a job search is clearly as much an art as it is a science. There are no clear-cut "5-step plans" for capturing a position. However, taking the time to do those little extras will enhance your chances considerably, moving you up the bell curve of opportunity with each step taken. The cream rises to the top, a process that will only make us stronger as a profession. Make certain you're part of that cream!

References
1. MacKay H. *Dig Your Well Before You're Thirsty.* New York, NY: Doubleday; 1997.
2. Krannich CR, Krannich RL. *Dynamite Networking for Dynamite Jobs.* Manassas Park, Va: Impact Publications; 1996.
3. Peters T. *The Circle of Innovation.* New York, NY: Vintage Books; 1999.
4. Ailes R. *You Are the Message.* New York, NY: Doubleday; 1995.

Just Look at Yourself

Stuck in the Middle?

You needn't stay wedged between the entry level and the executives. The key to moving forward? Physical therapist, evaluate and treat thyself.

"It is not a disgrace not to reach for the stars, but it is a disgrace to have no stars to reach for. Not failure, but low aim is a sin."

—Benjamin E Mayes[1]

There's no question that we've become a nation of "free agents." We read daily of executives leaving established companies for more lucrative opportunities. For those in entry-level clerical positions, there always seems to be a better option around the corner, offering more-attractive hours or higher pay.

But what about us? When the market for physical therapists is wide-open, there always seems to be a better offer in town if our current employer doesn't live up to its commitments. But what about when the market is tight? Are we stuck in the middle, between the entry level and the executives, with no option but to stick it out?

Of course not! Aim high! Reach for your goals! But before you can pursue that next position (or your first position, if you're just getting started), you need to take the same steps you take with your patients and clients.

The Evaluation

Tom Peters, in his outstanding book *The Brand You 50*,[2] offers up several questions that are tough to beat (and even tougher to answer) when it comes to evaluating your current "brand equity." What you must realize is that just as Coca-Cola and Maytag have substantial value (or equity) tied to their good name, so do you! The more valuable your brand, the more options you'll have as a therapist.

So let's get started with the evaluation. Fill in the blanks in the following statements:

I am known for _____
(list 2 to 4 things).

By this time next year, I plan also to be known for _____
(list 1 or 2 additional things).

Those aren't easy questions to start with, are they? You're a therapist, but what is it that you're *known for*? Do you have a niche that makes you stand out from most other therapists—such as a specialty in vestibular rehab, manual therapy, or lymphedema management? Do you teach? Have you built a solid network with physicians and the community? Do you feel you should perhaps be commanding a higher salary, given your experience and level of expertise?

And what about the future? Have you thought about what else you *plan* to be known for? Unfortunately, most people haven't. But it's critical that you consider what you're known for and what you plan to be known for before you can test the market for your skills.

Some of the ways in which my current project is challenging me are _____
(list 1 to 3 ways).

You're not encountering any challenges? Then there's no growth. We explain the "use it or lose it" principle to clients all the time, but then many of us come to work and do the same thing every day. Try to look for challenges instead. There's hardly a director or administrator alive who wouldn't love to have you step up to take on a new program or another project. In fact, it's very likely the *lack* of challenge in your position that's causing you to look around in the first place.

In the last 90 days I've learned _____
(list 1 to 3 new things).

Whether you're a recent grad or someone with a couple of decades of experience, your answer to this statement is critical! Far too many "experienced" therapists (the way they'd describe themselves because they've treated patients for many years) turn out not to have 15 years of experience, but rather 1 year of experience repeated 15 times. Hopefully this doesn't describe you. If it does, though, you need to make some changes.

Important new additions to my Rolodex in the last 90 days include _____ (list 2 to 4 names).

I discussed the importance of networking in "The 'Other' Net" (see page 10), but it can't be emphasized enough. If you have no network, your career isn't going to go anywhere. If you're content being a technician in your profession and have no problem with the idea of coming in and doing the same thing day after day for the rest of your working life, then you needn't worry too much about making contacts. (Of course, if you were that type of person you probably wouldn't be reading this article.)

But if you're seeking a profession (as opposed to being content to simply hold a job), you need to sit down today and figure out what opportunities are available to build and expand your network. Then *grow* for it! (Sorry—I couldn't resist.)

My public (local/regional/national/global) "visibility program" consists of _____ (list 1 or 2 things).

Heightening your visibility could include pursuing public speaking opportunities at obvious and even not-so-obvious venues. You'd be surprised what you can gain, for instance, from speaking to a group of elementary school kids—in terms of making connections with school administrators, teachers, and parents, and boosting your confidence for addressing higher-profile organizations down the road. (Never mind what Arnold Schwarzenegger went through in the movie *Kindergarten Cop*. Speaking before young children really isn't that tough, and you'll find that they'll laugh at almost every one of your jokes.) Consider bringing a handout with you—a self-screening for a specific dysfunction, or even a sample home health exercise for something like a sprained ankle. In addition to being educational, it'll enhance awareness of you and your organization.

Additional speaking opportunities could include contacting your community college or local civic organizations and clubs to provide an adult learning program, or approaching the physical therapy education program in your area. If you have a compelling message and deliver it with passion, people will listen.

Expanding your visibility through writing is another great option. This may mean sending an article to your state physical therapy newsletter or even to *PT—Magazine of Physical Therapy*, or simply keeping in written contact with old classmates from your physical therapy education program, politicians, and others in your network. And don't underestimate the power of a hand-written note in this age of word processing! The extra effort will stand out.

Another excellent way to increase your visibility and network with your peers (and grow in your profession at the same time) is to attend APTA's Annual Conference and the Association's Combined Sections Meeting. And think about joining a local APTA committee. There are lots of opportunities out there, but your eyes must be open before you can see—and seek—them. Again, you can plod along without making any additional effort, but even a small investment of time in some of these pursuits can pay off big in the long run in terms of growth and contacts.

My résumé/CV is discernably different from how it appeared at this time last year because I've _____
(list 1 or 2 noteworthy indicators of professional growth and/or standing in the past 12 months).

Has your résumé really changed in the past 12 months? Please consider the word "discernably." I'm not talking about a single, brief course you took. I'm referring to a new program you helped develop, new responsibilities you took on, a promotion you gained, a *series* of courses you took that have *significantly* enhanced your skills. And what are you doing now to enhance your résumé over the next 90 days?

The Treatment

Now that you've undergone evaluation by answering each tough question in turn—gaining in the process a better understanding of where you are and where you want to be in your professional life, and also an edge in your next job interview—it's time for you to get yourself some "treatment."

Positional tolerance training. Ask yourself the following questions:

- How important are benefits to you? What types of benefits do you think are most important?
- Is salary more or less important than benefits?
- Is your *potential* salary more important to you than your starting base?
- How important do you consider things such as time off, freedom (including liberty from micromanagement and having real input on projects), and flexible scheduling?
- Are you willing to relocate?
- What are your long-term professional goals?

Your answers will help start you down a specific path. If, for example, you like a lot of flexibility and independence and are willing to sacrifice a consistent salary at a certain level for the potential of big payoffs, you may want to look into a sales position. While that's certainly not for everyone, doing sales for a rehab company may allow you to keep your hands in the patient-care arena 1 or 2 days a week while trying something new. By the same token, if your long-term goal is to move into more of a clinical specialist's role, you'll need to look into mentors, study groups, and continuing education.

Gait training. There's usually more than one way to get from point A to point B. Before jumping over the fence to get to that "greener grass," look over the map very closely. Many employees tend to jump ship before considering all their options—and all the consequences of their decision.

For example, let's say you work for a moderate-sized company and are looking for a change. Through your network, you've found out about an opportunity across town before it hit the paper. You interview and are offered the job for $2,500 more per year than you're making now. Do you take it? Perhaps. But before deciding, take everything into consideration. For instance, what's the vacation policy at the new place? (Maybe you've built up 3 weeks annual leave at your current job but would be going all the way back to one week—or none the first year—if you change jobs.) You need to assess, too, how the other benefits compare—medical/dental, 401(k), opportunity for stock purchase, etc.

One option you might not have considered seriously enough is making a change within your current organization. Unless you're dead set on leaving for one reason or another, it's worth looking into the various opportunities available to you with your current employer—both at your current location and at other company sites, if applicable (and if you wouldn't mind moving). If you're an all-star, as I describe the term in "Tendencies of an All-Star" (see page 81), you'll likely find that your employer and supervisors would rather get creative and find ways to hang onto you than to let you slip away.

Home exercise program. But let's say you've explored your options at your current workplace and you've decided you really need to move on. Where do you go now? Well, you need to begin with a little research. Classified advertisements can be a good place to start in terms of finding out what jobs are available, but an even better idea is to determine which company has the qualities and benefits you're looking for and then begin pursuing that employer through an informational interview.

The company may not currently have a position available. However, it's very likely that if you appear knowledgeable and eager in an informational interview and ask what it would take to secure a position with the company when there *is* an opening, they'll give you straight answers. And, if you successfully follow up on all their recommendations and keep them informed of your progress, you may move to the top of their list of candidates.

Simply requesting an informational interview makes you stand out—to an extent. But you'll really shine if you can show the employer during the interview that you've taken the time to do your homework. Preparation is critical. Resources such as the Internet, health care professional journals, and your network can be invaluable tools in helping you know your audience better. The more you've learned about the organization, the more impressive you'll appear to your interviewer.

Mentors or a career coach also can be valuable tools as you move through this process. We all tend to have tunnel vision when it comes to our own performance. A mentor or career coach can identify areas of weakness and ways to capitalize on your strengths, work with you on résumés and cover letters, guide you through mock interviews, and help you develop a plan for the future.

Plan. "Continue" won't work for you here—even if that's the standard word you use as you move through your daily patient notes! To be successful in the job search, you need a plan. Sit down and write out specific goals and how you're going to get there. Treat your job search like a job! Have a daily plan of attack that covers who you're going to contact, what you're going to do, how you're going to follow up, and when each step will be completed.

Accountability also is invaluable—you need someone who can be trusted with the confidential nature of your pursuit to hold you accountable. Often it's easy to rationalize delays in goal setting and laxness about meeting timetables unless you've got another person—whether a spouse, friend, coach, or mentor—pushing you.

Outcome. Whatever happens as a result of this entire process, you'll find it quite valuable in the long run. You'll learn more about yourself and the company for which you're working. You'll likely gain a greater understanding of the industry and the market, and you're certain to expand your network.

Don't settle. Aim high! Remember: If you aim for the stars and fall short—while others hesitate and remain earthbound—you're still likely to reach the moon!

References
1. cybernation.com. Available at www.cybernation.com/quotationcenter/quotelist.php?type=s. Accessed March 7, 2006.
2. Peters T. *The Brand You 50.* New York, NY: Alfred A Knopf; 1999.

Escape!

Want to enhance your business and advance professionally? Perhaps you should get away from it all. Here's how to do retreats right.

You have 200 e-mail messages, 35 voicemail messages, 15 faxes, and dozens of phone calls to answer in addition to your daily workload. In the midst of all this, your management team is expected to come up with brilliant ways to expand the business, build staff morale, and enhance customer service. While I hate to be the one to break the news to you, here's a little observation: It's *not* going to happen.

That doesn't mean it *can't* happen. But it certainly won't happen in that setting. Most managers get a few minutes at best to address most items in their daily schedule, but it takes much longer than that to give most matters the attention they truly deserve. That's why I'm a big proponent of taking 1- or 2-day retreats to recharge the team and get everyone pointed in the right direction.

While "getting away" sounds easy enough, you'll find that it actually takes an incredible amount of preparation and planning to do it right and achieve optimal results. You're well aware (I hope!) of how long it takes to prepare for a well-run hour-long meeting. Well, planning for and facilitating even a one-day retreat requires a real commitment. Believe me, though, it's time well spent.

Getting Started

The biggest single mistake I find managers making when it comes to retreats is not being clear about purpose. If a client walked in your door, one of your first questions likely would be, "How may we help you?" If the client's response was, "I want to improve," but she couldn't pinpoint *what* she wanted to improve (function? strength? range of motion?), you'd have a much more difficult time bringing value to the interaction. But often managers schedule a retreat—having heard how great they can be—and later realize that they've never really identified the event's purpose. What do you hope to achieve? Here are a few typical purposes of retreats:

- To build a more cohesive team,
- To solve a specific challenge or combination of challenges,
- To create a new business plan,

- To help change the organization's focus (for example, strengthening its entrepreneurial base), and
- To offer everyone an opportunity to catch up on their discharge notes. (Okay, maybe not!)

The design of a retreat focused on building teamwork will be very different from the design of one focused on solving a number of challenges. But until you've determined your primary purpose, don't attempt to do anything more, because this decision will drive all of your future ones.

The Budget (Time and $$)

Once you've determined your retreat's purpose, it's time to assess how much you want to spend, both timewise and in dollars and cents. Ask the following questions as you begin the assessment process:

- How many (and which) people should attend?
- Should it be 1 or 2 days?
- Should you hold it in or out of town?
- Should you prepare your meal or meals there, have them catered, or go to a restaurant?
- Should you use an outside facilitator?
- Should there be entertainment?
- What should be on the agenda?

With a little creativity it's easy to keep costs reasonable. For example, our neighborhood has a beautiful facility that costs less than $150 a day for area residents. While that won't work for an overnight retreat, it's perfect for a single-day event, and it's great on the budget. If you plan your retreat far enough in advance and can be a little flexible, many hotels offer special deals on meeting rooms during their off-peak times.

Entertainment can cost big bucks, but again, with a little creativity—and an adventurous group—you can have a great time at little or no cost. Activities such as taking a hike or playing Frisbee golf can be as enjoyable as something pricey.

Supplies

Even if you're going to have the event catered or eat your meals out, there are many supplies you'll want to consider bringing along. I'll never live down forgetting to bring coffee to a 2-day mountain retreat! (I don't drink coffee, but obviously I'm in the minority.) Avoid my mistake by making a list and running it by a couple of people before making a trip to the store. Some common needs include tons of pens and pads of paper, poster board, music, Scotch/masking tape, snacks and drinks, and team-building materials. (More on that last need toward the end of this column.)

The Schedule

You've got your purpose and your budget in place. Now it's time to fill in the gaps, based on the choices you've made thus far. Here's a hint I've learned the hard way over the years, while organizing and facilitating many, many retreats: Don't pack too much into the schedule—and include some agenda items that can be eliminated on the fly if your team gets on a particularly productive jag. You'll likely, however, want to budget time for many of these activities:

- Travel to offsite events,
- Meals (including preparation time if they're not catered or you're not eating out),
- Group discussions,
- Team-building activities (separate from or as a part of breaks),
- Group breakout sessions,
- Personal reflection on the day's events,
- Presentations by attendees,
- Entertainment and outdoor activities, and
- De-briefing/wrap-up/closing survey.

Once your schedule is set, it's time for the specific preparation. If, for example, the retreat's primary purpose is to build a closer team, a tool such as the Myers-Briggs Type Indicator (MBTI) can be an invaluable aid to understanding the temperaments and tendencies of your various team members, and to facilitating better teamwork in the long term. To gain the full benefit of the MBTI, however, it must be administered by a certified MBTI career consultant. You can pick up some of the basics about the MBTI through such resources as *Please Understand Me II*[1] by David Keirsey.

Another way to prepare people for the retreat might be to give them a book or audiotape to review up to a month in advance. If the retreat is to focus primarily on leadership, for example, books such as Stephen Covey's *Principle-Centered Leadership*[2] or Warren Bennis's *Leaders*[3] are of reasonable length and are ideal for group discussion.

Ground Rules

Setting ground rules is a *critical* but often-forgotten step. Most people's tendency, unfortunately, is to lean toward the negative. In a retreat setting, where people have a chance to let their hair down, allowing negative comments to dominate the conversation can spell disaster for even the best-planned retreat. (Believe me—I've made the mistake of letting it happen!) That doesn't mean conversation must be kept at a superficial level, though. Rather, make it clear to attendees that the focus will be on the positive, and that when negatives do arise the emphasis will be on finding solutions, not just letting things slide into a complaint session. This is not a Disney movie. Candor, honesty, and open discussion are valuable and important, as long as the focus stays centered on finding solutions. Don't bend on this issue! Having an experienced facilitator on hand can help keep things on track, but stating your goal of positive discussion before the retreat ever takes place makes a big difference. I've even gone to the extent of telling prospective attendees to stay home if they don't plan on going into the retreat with good mental posturing.

Other ground rules should include fighting fair—participants will no doubt get into some arguments, but disagreements should never be allowed to get personal—and coming in prepared, with advance reading done and presentations ready to go. Also, establish at the outset that, while you'll be debating a variety of issues on which there will be differences of opinion, once the team reaches agreement, everyone will unite behind those decisions.

Team Building

Regardless of the retreat's primary purpose, it's likely that enhanced team building is one outcome you're seeking. Many books and Web sites provide team-building ideas and exercises, but let me get you started with one of my favorites.

- *Goal:* As a team, build a structure that will "catch" an egg dropped from a height of at least 8 feet without breaking it. If you have more than 5 people, consider splitting into smaller groups and competing to see which team can build the structure that can successfully catch the egg from the greatest height.
- *Supplies:* Each team will need a box of straws, a roll of masking tape, a dozen eggs, and some plastic to lay down under the structures.
- *Time:* This can vary, but 30 minutes should be more than adequate to build the structure.

This simple exercise stretches the imagination, gets the competitive juices flowing, and gets the team working together. It's also very easy to tie the different portions of this exercise into your theme, given a little creativity. For example, you can tie building the structure to developing a new program or programs. Then you can convey the idea that, just as the structure protects the egg, the new program protects the staff against downturns in other parts of your business.

Debriefing/Survey

Keep it simple. One of the easiest ways to wrap things up is to use a "stop-start-continue" exercise in which you ask retreat participants for specifics in each category:

- *Stop:* What they would eliminate from the retreat, and why.
- *Start:* What they'd like to see added to retreats in the future.
- *Continue:* What they felt went well and should be a part of future retreats.

This is an easy way to get on-the-spot feedback that can improve the next retreat immensely. I typically encourage people to plan two retreats each year. Suggestions generated from one event can be implemented in the next one.

Holding a successful retreat requires a great deal of preparation and planning. But if you're seeking a way to stretch your team, improve performance, enhance your leadership skills, and/or create a brainstorming blowout, getting away may be just what you need to step it up to the next level!

References
1. Keirsey D. *Please Understand Me II: Temperament, Character, Intelligence.* Del Mar, Calif: Prometheus Nemesis Book Co; 1998.
2. Covey S. *Principle-Centered Leadership.* New York, NY: Fireside; 1992.
3. Bennis W, Nanus B. *Leaders: Strategies for Taking Charge.* New York, NY: HarperBusiness; 1997.

Lessons Learned Along the Road

Reflections on an entrepreneurial career, with some questions that physical therapists ought to consider.

Okay, I admit it: I've always had a thing for entrepreneurship. That doesn't mean I've always been successful in entrepreneurial pursuits, however. I began establishing my own little businesses at age 8 and have been at it ever since. Some of them did quite well; others failed miserably. Both my struggles and my successes have taught me some important lessons. I'd like to share a few of them with you in hopes that they may strike a chord for you in your professional pursuits.

Sticks on the Street Corner

My first entrepreneurial pursuit—that I can remember, anyway—consisted of attempting to sell carved wooden sticks at the four-way stop near our house. My little brother, you see, had been carving very small, simple sticks into little arrows and selling them for 10 cents each and actually had been quite successful at it (yes, entrepreneurship runs in my family). I figured if he could sell his sticks for a dime, I could come out with a larger, fancier version and sell them for $5 or more apiece.

So I went to work, carving sticks by the hour and eventually setting up my own stand. The problem was, my little brother had carved himself quite a niche serving kids with little money and adults who took pity on the little 6-year-old businessman and were willing to spare a dime to keep him from getting discouraged.

My product addressed neither of those markets. Kids couldn't afford to pay $5 for a carved wooden stick, and adults, to be honest, were loath to shell out that kind of money to an older kid who wasn't quite as cute as my younger brother. I struck out—completely! All those hours of carving and not even a single sale! But I did get my first bit of insight into a key of successful entrepreneurship.

Lesson learned: Minimize overhead through bootstrapping (building success from a small initial investment). Instead of spending hours preparing multiple products for sale, I should have carved just a couple of sample items, done some test marketing, then moved on or made adjustments. Instead, I was stuck with a pile of unnecessary, unused, and undesirable inventory. Fortunately, it was inventory that cost me only time rather than money, but I suffered for days from the blisters I got from all that carving!

Food for thought:

- What program could I start in my clinic for, say, $2,500? Where would I spend the money?
- What could I initiate if I had just $1,000? What would be my priority then?
- How about if I had just $500?

Gum Up for Grabs

I took my stick experiences to heart and next moved into another area—gum sales. On the way to junior high school I would stop by the 7-11 and purchase a pack of gum (eventually several packs) for 25 cents. Each pack contained five individually wrapped pieces. Once at school, I would turn around and sell each stick of gum for 25 cents, providing an instant 500% return on my investment.

I would then reinvest this return in additional inventory (after feeding my addiction to football cards). My "company" grew at a rate that would soon be the envy of any of today's "Inc 500" list of overachieving small businesses. Unfortunately, however, the principal eventually informed me that this type of profit-making was not allowed at school. While I promptly shut down my operation, I had felt the thrill of my first successful (if short) entrepreneurial endeavor.

Lessons learned: 1) High margins are a good thing! With just a small investment, strong profit margins that are pumped back into a product or service offering can add up quickly. In addition, supply and demand can work wonders for such margins. (Especially when kids are spending their parents' money in most cases!) The caveat that I also learned, however, is that *2) **for long-term success, you have to play by the rules!***

Food for thought:

- Are you focusing your energies on programs that have the highest possible margins? If not, is there a compelling reason why you're not, or have you gotten sidetracked and lost your entrepreneurial edge?
- Are there instances in which you've played outside the rulebook that could endanger your long-term success? If so, what do you plan to do about it?

Lawns With a Loaner

With my gum business shut down, my radar went up for the "next big thing." It turned out to be right in my own front yard—promising me dollars, not quarters, as long as I was willing to invest a little sweat equity.

There were plenty of lawns on my street that needed mowing, so I made a business deal with my dad: I'd do our lawn for pennies if I could use his mower for my business. I was set! For the next 3 years, I mowed up to seven lawns per week during the growing season, earning enough money to eventually buy my own car at 16.

Lesson learned: Partnerships often provide a valuable way to keep overhead down, increasing profit margins.

Food for thought:

- With whom (or with what programs) could you partner inside your organization to enhance growth and limit overhead?
- What outside partners might you consider?

Consultant at 16

At 16, with my lawn business passed on to my younger brother, I set out to enter the "real world" of work. I was surprised by what I saw. As a bagger at the local grocery store, I got a charge out of trying to keep up with three checkers simultaneously. At the same time, however, I saw fellow employees competing to see how little work they could get by with in an 8-hour shift. I was there to earn a paycheck—not get a handout!—but it was clear to me that that wasn't the prevailing attitude among my fellow workers.

In fact, I was so driven to earn an honest buck that I still remember the look of shock on the manager's face when he offered to let me go home 25 minutes early one day. With a quick calculation, I figured out that 25 minutes would cost me about $2.10 and responded, "That's okay. I'd rather stay, if someone else would like to take off." (The manager quickly found another taker.)

It was at the same store that I got my first taste for consulting. After a few weeks on the job, I went home and typed up a multi-page report on all the ways in which I felt we could improve the store. (Remember, I was 16 at the time and relatively clueless about business, sales, etc.) With butterflies in my stomach, I slipped the report—my name clearly written on the front—under the manager's door.

A few minutes later the ominous-sounding words "Brad Cooper, please come to the manager's office" were blaring over the loudspeaker. (Hearing such a request with one's name attached to it was not typically a positive thing.) But the manager was charitable enough to at least pretend that he was taking me seriously. While he probably laughed privately at my presumption, he kept the passion burning in this young entrepreneur by playing along. And who knows—maybe there really was a good idea in there somewhere.

Lesson learned: Don't quench the fire of dreamers. I've been in that manager's position many times since then, and I always think of him and the respect that he showed me. So, I'm not about to be responsible for dousing the flame of initiative in an energetic innovator. At worst, I'll gently offer another perspective and close the discussion with a comment along the lines of, "But in reality, it's the passion of the program's champion—not the plan itself—that often determines success or failure."

Food for thought:

- You managers out there—do you put more stock in the plan or the person?
- You "dreamers" out there—if you're the champion of a new program, do you wait until the plan is perfect or do you get the ball rolling and make adjustments along the way?

If You Build It They May Not Come

Two master's degrees, several business pursuits, and about 15 years later, I started up a company called TheraCoach. Begun at a time when jobs in our profession were very hard to come by, the company was designed to provide day-long or multiple-day programs that associations and corporations would sponsor for their members on how to secure a job in physical therapy or make best use of their skills. I put together a board of directors, manuals, handouts, and a presentation. We picked our office site, bought a mailing list, and sent out flyers—expending many hours and hundreds of dollars in the process.

Then we waited by the phone and the mailbox for the onslaught of responses that were sure to come. One week went by. Then 2. Then a month, 2 months. Nothing! Not a single response! (Some of our flyers came back marked "Return To Sender," but we didn't figure those "responses" counted.) Ouch!

I later revamped the company to focus more on one-on-one coaching, while concentrating on corporate clients to expand my speaking business. But that experience proved a tough—and expensive—one to go through.

Lesson learned: If you build it, there's no guarantee that they really will come! Be careful about putting all of your eggs in one basket—even when the basket looks failsafe!

Food for thought:

- Who are the managers who believe in you and your program?
- Who should you take to lunch and otherwise cultivate to try to secure the long-term business you'll need to be successful?

Keep on Learning

All of this brings me to my current status as a speaker and consultant in the areas of team-building, sales, leadership, and customer service. I never would have had a chance of success had I not benefited so greatly from the lessons I learned along the way. Nor will the business continue to grow unless my learning continues. Here are some great ways, I've found, to keep learning:

- *Form mentor groups.* Picking the brains of other physical therapists (PTs) in private practice is not just a good idea, it's a requirement. Success is often about leverage; by sharing ideas with others on a regular basis, you will leverage your potential much more quickly than you would by sticking to yourself. *Ask yourself: Who could I invite today to join with me in a monthly or quarterly brainstorming and support group?*

- *Go to the pros!* I'm a pretty darn good speaker but I don't write computer code, so I invest my time in customizing the programs I offer and enhancing my speaking skills, while hiring others to design my Web site, market my materials, and edit my tapes and books. Discover what you do well and focus your time there. Look over your daily schedule. *Do you consistently give yourself the time and opportunity to do the things that you do well? If not, rearrange things and make it so!*

- *Go to the pros again!* While I've found my niche as a speaker, I must continue to improve if I'm going to compete for the top-level (and top-dollar) keynote addresses. To do so means working with the best coaches in the industry, in terms of both technique and business plan development. Are you doing the same? Whether you're looking to move to the next level in clinical skills or management strategies or professional development, ask around for the names of the best in the business. Contact them and make an investment in your future. *What professional courses do you plan to take this year? How are you developing your skills as a manager?*

- *Get involved with your professional association.* If you want to get the most out of your professional potential, invest time and money in getting to know and learning from people who share your goals and are headed in the same direction as you. In our case as PTs, that means stepping up to the plate for our professional association, APTA. Have you re-upped for next year? Have you gotten involved in your local chapter? *Also, are there organizations you should consider joining in addition to APTA, such as the American College of Healthcare Executives, or Toastmasters?*

Developing as a successful professional in health care management requires focus, time, and learning through trial and error. Ask the tough questions regularly and be willing to fail on occasion. You'll likely find yourself learning important lessons along the way and will see yourself rise to new heights!

Where's the Passion?

Do you feel as if you're dragging in your professional life? Here are some ways to bring back that loving-it feeling.

Solid clinical skills, an extensive knowledge base, years of experience, and exceptional people skills: You can have all of that and still be lacking a critical component of excellence—passion.

You remember passion, don't you? Think about when you first started out as a clinician: You probably felt a little nervous and in need of seasoning, yet certain that in the long run you would make a difference. You knew that you had a lot of hard work ahead of you, but you were ready to set the world of physical therapy on fire—to change lives, maybe even change the profession.

Over time, however, perhaps the passion dwindled. Maybe your sense of clarity faded about why you were there and what you were destined to accomplish—buried in seemingly endless stacks of paperwork, a bulging appointment book, and an ever-growing collection of insurance regulations.

In his book *Wild at Heart*,[1] John Eldredge tells readers: "Don't ask yourself what the world needs. Ask yourself what makes you come alive, and go do that, because what the world needs is people who have come alive."

Does reading those words make you smile, because your professional pursuits do, indeed, make you feel alive? Or does Eldredge's challenge make you want to run and hide, because it reminds you that your work doesn't enliven you the way it used to?

If your response is the latter, I'm here to tell you that it doesn't have to be that way! You can rediscover that which makes your heart jump. Here are some tips for getting started:

Step back. The first step toward getting back on track in reclaiming your passion as a clinician (and perhaps, too, as a leader on whose actions the livelihoods of other PTs and PTAs depend) is to ask yourself what percentage of your work day fits into each of the following categories:

- Category I: "Wow, I *love* this stuff!"
- Category II: "It's okay; I can tolerate it."
- Category III: "I *hate* this part."

How does your typical day at the clinic stack up? Some of the physical therapy leaders with whom I work in my workshops and seminars place almost none of their work day in Category I. In fact, just recently, a leader who's known to her colleagues and patients for her passion and energy told me that 100% of her activities now fit into Category II. No wonder she confides that she finds herself drained and unfulfilled in her profession.

How about you? Do you get up in the morning eagerly anticipating the day ahead, or do you wish you could just stay in bed? If you can't honestly say that you spend at least 15% to 30% of your day at the clinic in Category I, it's time for you to re-prioritize, re-analyze, and revamp your professional life.

Step out. If you've determined that you spend a negligible percentage of any given day at the clinic in Category I, the next question you should ask yourself is, will you be satisfied with spending most of your working hours this year wishing and waiting for the day to end? If not, consider adopting some or all of the following steps—each of which can help shake you out of the doldrums and reenergize your professional life:

- *Start a journal.* Taking just a few minutes each week to jot down your on-the-job (or off-the-job) thoughts can do a couple of very good things. For one thing, it can help you discern patterns of thought and behavior and prompt you to brainstorm some great ideas for positive change. I've kept a journal for years. I keep it handy at home and in my carry-on bag when I'm traveling. Whenever I'm particularly discouraged, or in the midst of a brainstorm, I pull out my journal and keep the pen moving. The left side of the page is where brainstorms go—ideas for retreats, training programs, and new business. The right side of the page is where I simply record what I'm thinking and feeling. Reviewing these notes weeks or months later often lends a new perspective to the path ahead.

  The other positive about keeping a journal? You may find that the process of writing about your experiences in the clinic helps mitigate some of the stress related to them.

- *Check your "balance meter"*—the weight you give and the amount of time you devote to your professional life, as opposed to your outside pursuits. By "outside pursuits," I mean:

  Physical. You preach physical fitness to your patients and clients, but do you devote sufficient time to physical activity in your own life? You needn't find a marathon to run—even walking during your lunch hour a few days a week can refresh your mind and your body, giving you extra energy to tap at the clinic.

  Social. Take a moment to jot down the names of the three to six people closest to you. If you were to ask each of them to assess how much you care about them based on your actions, words, and attention over the past 6 months, what would they say?

Spiritual. Is your spiritual life important to you? If so, would a casual observer be able to tell? If not, have you considered further exploring your spiritual side and making it a more vibrant part of your everyday life?

Financial. Have you dug yourself into a financial hole? Did you make an ill-advised decision to buy a new car, rather than a used one? Did you purchase a house that's bigger—and more expensive—than what you needed? Has a bad financial decision from the past boxed you into having to work an extra job, put in a lot of overtime, or remain with an employer you'd prefer to leave behind? How much money will you need for retirement? Do you have any idea? Stop kidding yourself that "everything will work out." Maybe it will—but only if you take some steps to make financial prosperity possible in the real world!

- *Form your own "mastermind" team.* Hook up with a group of four to six professional peers whose goals and dreams are similar to your own, and meet as a group for a couple of hours each month. Use that time to mastermind ideas, share your progress, and hold each other responsible for pursuing your goals. This can be a powerful vehicle for gaining new ideas and building accountability into your professional life.

> Hook up with a group of four to six professional peers whose goals and dreams are similar to your own, and meet as a group for a couple of hours each month.

- *Give back.* It's amazing how good our own life appears when we look away from ourselves and toward opportunities to help those around us, beyond the clinic. For example, early in my physical therapy career, I worked part time as the junior and high school youth director at our local church. In that role, I had an opportunity to take several high school kids to Ecuador on a mission trip. The result (both for me and for the students) was a new perspective on how good we have it here in the States. Our "problems" don't quite stack up beside life-and-death dilemmas such as not having enough food to eat or clean water to drink. When I returned home I stopped griping about many of the little things that had upset me and found renewed energy in making the best of the amazing opportunities before me.

Don't wait! Just as it's inadvisable for people who need the services of a PT to put off the visit for an extra month, so, too, is any delay in trying to rejuvenate yourself professionally likely to be counterproductive. The more you delay, the more difficult change promises to become.

Step forward. Take time to re-prioritize and think about why you're doing what you're doing. It's amazing what clarity of purpose can do for someone who's dragging his or her feet.

Have you ever conducted a priority check? Write down the 16 activities that take up the greatest amount of your time and energy at the clinic. What are the top two or three things on that list? Are there several activities farther down on that roster that energize you much more than the first few items do? If so, could you reorganize your work schedule so that you could spend the majority of your time doing the things that invigorate you? The answer, for everyone, is yes. The profession of physical therapy once excited you. Rearranging your day can help bring the excitement back.

That's what happened to me. After having spent several years as a health care manager, I found myself dragging my body into work. My wife (a side note—pay attention to those who know you best when they make caring suggestions) reminded me of how my eyes always lit up whenever I had an opportunity to see leaders develop. She suggested that I plan a management retreat and get back to meeting with my team members individually to help them develop their leadership skills. I took her advice, and quickly found that the renewed energy I felt spilled over to my other tasks and priorities. In fact, a passion for leadership, patient care, and life often derives from clarity of mission. Make the time to create that clarity, and life will never be the same.

Leaders, current and future, come in all shapes and sizes, from a variety of backgrounds, and with a range of goals for the future. But one trait common to all effective leaders is that they know in their gut that what they're doing makes a difference. They're committed to making things happen. And that requires passion. Without passion, there's a gaping hole in the day that activities and strategic plans simply can't fill.

Got passion? If not, think back on when you did, and know that you can get it back. It may be time for you to take a good look at yourself. There's a leader in the mirror, staring back at you, and it's well within your means to free that individual from the lethargy that's holding him or her (you!) back.

Reference
1. Eldredge J. *Wild at Heart: Discovering the Secret of a Man's Soul*. Nashville, Tenn: Thomas Nelson, Inc; 2001.

What's Your "Fear Factor"?

Facing your fears can help you achieve your professional goals—and you don't have to walk on glass or take a snake bath.

Is fear of the unknown keeping you from doing everything you know you must do to meet your professional goals and/or advance your career? What is a physical therapist (PT) or physical therapist assistant (PTA) to do?

I wouldn't blame anyone for choosing not to eat putrefied meat or jump into a shark tank on TV's "Fear Factor"—the small screen's version of reality—but when it comes to achieving professional fulfillment in your own real life, avoidance isn't the answer. Let me illustrate that conviction with some personal examples.

In the wee hours of a Sunday morning last November, I was one of the few successful registrants (if you can call 1,000 "a few") for the Escape from Alcatraz Triathlon in San Francisco. Registration opened at 1 am and closed at 2:45 am, with many thousands of athletes missing the cut. When registration ended, I was happy and my wife was perplexed by the number of very strange people who had chosen to forgo a night's sleep for this "privilege."

After experiencing the initial thrill of making the cut, I headed back to bed, planning on getting some sleep. It didn't happen. For 2 hours I tossed and turned, suddenly realizing what I'd done. I would be starting off this race by jumping off a boat near Alcatraz Island into 55-degree water and swimming 1.5 miles in strong currents—with the possibility of meeting the occasional 2-ton sea lion along the way! And then I'd still have to complete the grueling bike and running segments of the race. Scared? You betcha!

But then I began thinking about some of the other things in my life that I'd found a little (or very) frightening at the time, and how each had eventually worked out:

- Asking Suzanna to marry me. Would she say yes? Could we really make a go of it for the long haul? What would the future hold for this naïve couple? (She said yes; we recently celebrated our 10th anniversary.)

- Giving my first big speech. What was I doing there? Would anyone actually come? Would they stay for the whole thing? (I survived, and nobody walked out.)

- The birth of our first child—and the second and the third. Would they be healthy? Could I provide for their needs? Was there hope for their future given all the uncertainty in the world? (They've turned out to be the coolest kids in the world—not that I'm prejudiced, of course!)

- The kickoff of my Champions Roundtable leadership retreat. Should I really attempt this just because it was a dream of mine? Was it really worth the 200 hours of preparation, when I didn't even know if people would attend? (It turned out to be one of the most exciting things I've ever been a part of.)

You get the idea. It seemed that for every single example that came to mind, the result proved to be life-changing in an extremely positive way. And I found that, in each case, my fear actually had been beneficial—it had prompted me to assess, reassess, and plan, increasing my chances of ultimate success.

Currently, swimming is my weakest event in the triathlon. But it won't be for much longer! I've joined a masters swim club in order to improve my stroke and endurance—and that's something I would not have done without the motivation of the extremely demanding Alcatraz event. Now, how about you? Have you found a way to turn your fears into springboards to achievement?

When it comes to our careers as PTs and PTAs, we, like so many people, easily can become complacent. Consider your answers to the following questions:

- In what ways are you trying to expand your skills beyond their current range? Have you undergone, or even considered, management training? Have you looked into developing new programs at your clinic? Have you tried to learn more about how to market your practice?

- What project might you take on this year that would be of significant value to your employer, or your clinic if you're the owner, and also would enhance your résumé?

- In what ways do you plan to expand your clinical knowledge in the next 12 months?

- Who are your mentors? When was the last time you connected with them over breakfast or paid them visits to get their feedback on your professional pursuits?

- Who are *you* mentoring?

Many of the things that stretch us professionally are the very same things that stretch us beyond our comfort zones. That's why they're not easy. But they're worth it!

Risk Is Relative

What about when things don't go smoothly? It's not so hard to stretch yourself when everything goes according to plan. But that doesn't always happen, does it?

As a writer, speaker, and career coach, I tend to focus on the positive. That might suggest to some people that, in my own life, things always have gone just the way I hoped and envisioned they would. Not so! Let's revisit the examples I mentioned earlier:

- Asking Suzanna to marry me. She did say yes ... but then she had second thoughts, and we really questioned whether we were right for each other. We tied the knot only after nearly a year of prayer, discussions, and contemplation. That was one of the toughest years of my life, wondering what was going to happen.

- Giving my first big speech. While it's true that nobody walked out that time (maybe they all felt sorry for me!), that doesn't mean it never happens. I've seen my share of people head for the door in the years since. I always tell myself, "They're leaving for a good reason—not because they're bored with my speech," but it's never easy to watch.

- The birth of our children. We've been so fortunate with them; I'm one proud daddy! As any parent knows, though, there have been and will continue to be many anxious moments and heartaches along the way. There's no choice but to be strong and deal with it all.

- The kickoff of my Champions Roundtable leadership retreat. That first one was very successful and exciting, but registration for the following one was so slow that I had to push back the date. Deflating? Yes!

The point is, every one of those things proved well worth the risks and the inevitable setbacks and disappointments along the way. You may be tempted to think that there's no harm in staying on the same track and just letting things happen, but isn't sitting still at least as risky—if not riskier—than moving forward into unknown territory? How many people do you know whose professional skills have stagnated and whose careers have stalled because they haven't addressed and conquered the challenges and fears that confront them?

Release the Butterflies

When I was growing up, my mom often repeated the adage "no risk, no gain." Not only have I taken her advice to heart throughout my life, but I also have found from firsthand experience that the bigger the risk you take on, the better you ensure that you're prepared to meet it.

In other words, the bigger the stretch, the stronger the jump-start. So, when was the last time you took a risk big enough to send the butterflies fluttering in your stomach? When was the last time you stretched yourself far enough that you couldn't rely on your existing skills and needed to acquire new ones? When was the last time you moved past your comfort zone—and into the danger zone?

Consider this point, too: Taking risks doesn't always ensure success, but it does ensure that you're truly alive inside. Does it really matter if you live to be 102 if you look back on a lifetime of inaction and regret? Maybe it's time to take another look at a challenge from which you once shrank and put your own personal fear factor to work for you.

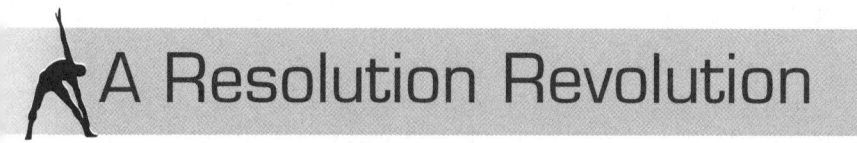

A Resolution Revolution

Don't give up on your New Year's goals. Together, we can make them happen.

Let me just cut to the chase and ask you this: How many of you entered the new year with a self-improvement resolution or two at least on your mind, if not set down on paper for loved ones to see, or spoken aloud in front of witnesses? Can I see a show of hands?

Just as I thought. I see a lot of hands.

Now, with the new year only a month old, how many of those resolutions already have gone the way of those Christmas trees that stood so tall only a few weeks ago? Again, a show of hands?

Wow, I still see a lot of hands.

Every year, by the time the average person wakes up from the onslaught of trips to the mall and then back-to-back college football games, those resolutions already have fallen by the wayside. Why? Two reasons, primarily.

First, most people aren't really receptive to change. We naturally resist it. To cite just one example, if you're very young or have a short attention span, you may not remember "New Coke," which lasted in the marketplace for about a nanosecond several years ago. The Coca-Cola Company had conducted all manner of focus groups and consumer surveys, and the results were in: Americans overwhelmingly preferred the new flavor. The rollout was supported by millions upon millions of dollars worth of advertising, and it looked as if "old" Coke soon would be gone—yesterday's news.

When New Coke hit the shelves, however, you would've thought that the United States government had proposed that we change the colors in Old Glory! Coke drinkers went berserk! They would have nothing to do with the new formula. Within weeks, tried-and-true traditional Coke was back on the market—to stay. Change, even in something as seemingly innocuous as sugar water, was not to be tolerated.

The second reason our resolutions tend quickly to fail is that we seldom are fully invested in the outcome. We "want" to do this. We'd "like" to do that. But if we don't do it, well, there's always that show to watch on television tonight.

But what if you were to throw caution and inertia to the winds and commit yourself to making this the year you embrace change, put your foot down, draw a line in the sand, and say, "No more excuses. No more delays. No more saying, 'Someday.' I'm going to do it—now!" I can assure you it's not too late, either in this year or your life.

Ask Why

What's that thing you'd like to do "someday" to improve yourself, your family, and or your community? What about:

- Taking a trip to help rebuild an area in need (like the Southern Gulf region after Hurricane Katrina in 2005)?
- Signing up to take a specialist-certification exam?
- Running a marathon?
- Losing 50 pounds and becoming a role model for the high percentage of your patients who are overweight?
- Running for office in your APTA chapter?
- Putting out your cigarette for the last time and beginning the cleansing of your lungs?
- Volunteering to coach your daughter's hockey team?
- Joining your local church, synagogue, or mosque—as a committed member rather than merely as an occasional attendee?
- Beginning work on your transitional DPT?
- Sitting down with a financial planner and putting together a realistic budget that will get you out of debt—permanently?
- Asking that man or woman to marry you?

Maybe none of those examples fits your circumstances. But I'll bet there's something big—potentially life-changing, even—on which you've been chewing for a while. Maybe you've even made one or more abortive assaults on it already. Well, this time it's going to be different. We're going to work on it together. This time, we're going to make it happen!

How? We're going to take those two primary reasons why resolutions die and remove them from the picture altogether. First, the issue with change. Change can be overcome if you have a big enough "why." Had the Coca-Cola Company stated, "We've changed our formula because we're getting reports that the old formula is causing the index finger of Coke drinkers to fall off," I doubt anyone would have complained. Granted, lawsuits by index-fingerless Coke drinkers might well have put the company out of business, but consumers wouldn't have griped about the formula change itself.

What's your "why?" Is it big enough to provoke you to change your behavior or attitude enough to fulfill your resolution?

The second thing we're going to do is do this together. Go to www.apta.org/messageboards, click on "PT Mag Career Coach," and outline your goals for the year and your big, honkin', monstrously huge "whys." We'll compare notes and see how we're all progressing. We'll be an electronic support group for one another! Together, we'll get it done!

Are you in? I am. After years of dreaming about it and saying "someday," I recently signed up for my first Ironman Triathlon—a race that starts with a 2.4 mile swim, continues with a 112-mile bike ride, and wraps up with a marathon run (26.2 miles). I work out a lot, but I'm still a little nervous about this one. That's a long race!

So what's my big "why?" Yes, the event is something I've wanted to tackle for years, but with a busy family and professional life, desire alone isn't enough motivation for me to devote the combined 5,000 miles or so of swimming, cycling, and running I figure I'll need to log while training for the event. My big motivator, rather, is 40 kids in an orphanage in the Ukraine, for whom I'll be trying to raise $20,000 through the Janus Capital Group's Janus Charity Challenge. I'll know that every step, every stroke, every pedal will be making a difference in those kids' future. That's a huge why!

Make the Year Yours

Goal-achievement is an interesting thing. In many ways it's a matter of momentum. Achieve one big goal and going after the next one becomes easier. Run that first 10K and the idea of entering a marathon doesn't seem quite so scary. Knock out your debt and beginning a retirement fund becomes possible. For many of us, getting into physical therapy school (or through neurology class once there!) was the last really tough goal we pursued. Isn't it time we set our sights on a new one?

So what's it going to be? Another year of getting by? Another year of counting the days until the weekend? Another year of looking at someone or something from the outside and saying to yourself, "Someday I'd like to do that"?

Or is this going to be your year? The year you say to yourself and the world, "I'm in! Sign me up for something big!"

It's Your Attitude

Awakening the "WOW!"

Has physical therapy become just a job to you? Following this five-step rejuvenation plan will re-energize you and remind you why you joined the profession.

Do you remember a few years ago, when you had the passion—when you were thrilled to be a physical therapist (PT) or physical therapist assistant (PTA), and were excited to have the chance to make a difference in people's lives every day that you practiced, or taught, or conducted research? For many PTs and PTAs, what I call the "WOW! factor" still burns brightly. For others, however, physical therapy has become just a job. For those in the second category, here are five steps to reawaken your WOW!

Step One: Live "On Purpose"

Few people live "on purpose"—setting and pursuing specific goals. The vast majority of people live accidentally. Consider the comments you hear every day: "We'll just see what happens." "We'll take it as it comes." Even, "What can you do?" Do you hear the lack of purpose in those approaches to life? Those folks are living accidentally.

Any decent golfer knows very well the importance of picking a *specific* target, giving the mind an aiming point. The player's skill level may or may not allow him or her to deliver on the goal, but he or she will achieve better results by keeping a specific target in mind. Unfortunately, though, even those who know the value of applying this concept on the golf course typically neglect to do so in life.

Many people focus on what they *don't* want to have happen (ie, "I don't want to lose my job" or "I don't want to go into debt") instead of determining what they *do* want to happen. How about you? Every day you write out short- and long-term goals for your patients and plan your treatment around them. Have you done that for yourself lately? You would never drift through a series of treatment sessions without pursuing specific goals, right?

Start simple. Take a quick inventory of the following areas of your life and give yourself a rating from 1 to 5, with 5 equating to "couldn't be better" and 1 meaning "needs significant work":

- Relationships with family, coworkers, friends
- Professional growth
- Spiritual life
- Physical well-being
- Financial (ie, retirement) planning

How'd you do? Chances are, if your numbers are low, it's because you're living accidentally. Try living on purpose, however, and the results can be life-changing.

Take a simple example: financial planning. Many people are deeply in debt despite the strong economy and stock market. Certainly some of these folks have suffered some great misfortune that resulted in their indebtedness, but most simply let it happen, one day at a time, by overspending and neglecting to have a savings plan. But such plans needn't be elaborate: Do you realize that a 24-year-old person, saving just $5.47 a day (the cost of a trip to a fast-food restaurant) will have a million dollars at age 60 if he or she invests it wisely and receives a 12% return annually?

One other note about living on purpose: Accountability is critical. Just as your patients are more likely to perform their home exercise program when they know you're going to be checking up on them, you're much more likely to follow through on your plans when you've shared them with a friend, family member, or coworker who will hold you accountable.

Step Two: Get Back to the Basics

There are so many things in life over which you have no control, and upbringing and genetics obviously carry a great deal of weight in shaping who you are. However, such basics of life as fuel, sleep, and exercise are very much under your control, and their impact on the WOW! factor is incredibly significant.

Fuel. Pretend for a moment that you were to stake your life savings on the outcome of an auto race. The two competing cars were the exact same model, had the exact same engine, and were being driven by drivers with equal amounts of experience. The only difference was that car A had premium fuel and car B had second-rate fuel.

There's not a single person reading this column who wouldn't select car A, yet most people do just the opposite in their own lives, feasting on junk food. Don't get me wrong; I'm no nutritionist or health food fanatic. But I do know for certain that making a habit of eating smart—watching my fat intake, stocking up on fruits and vegetables, and otherwise adhering to a healthy diet— enhances my performance!

Here's a simple tip: Consider going nuts! More and more studies are showing that adding nuts (especially walnuts, almonds, and cashews) to your daily routine can reduce the incidence of heart disease, promote weight loss, and reduce your cancer risk.[1] And replacing that candy bar with a portion of nuts (just don't go overboard) will certainly help keep the motor running on all cylinders more consistently throughout the day!

Sleep. Most healthy adults need an average of 8 hours of sleep a night to function without sleepiness or drowsiness, but some individuals can get the same results with as little as 6 hours of sleep at night. Signs that you aren't getting enough sleep include irritability with others, difficulty concentrating or remembering facts, and trouble staying alert during boring or monotonous situations when fatigue often reveals itself.[2]

There are plenty of things you can do to better ensure that you get the amount of sleep you need to perform at your peak—things like avoiding caffeine, nicotine, and alcohol in the late afternoon and evening; getting regular exercise (more on that shortly); avoiding naps during the day if you have trouble sleeping at night; establishing a relaxing, regular bedtime routine; and making your sleep environment as comfortable, dark, and quiet as you can.[2]

Earlier this year, I made some conscious moves toward a better diet. I started reading the labels on breakfast cereals more closely (even the "healthy" brands tend to have hydrogenated fat and high-fructose corn syrup), I began bringing salads (often with tuna or salmon added) to work for lunch, and I started snacking on fruit or nuts during the day instead of candy or chips. At about the same time, I began trying to go to bed at about the same time every night. Ever since I made these changes, I've been sleeping better. In fact, I now find that I feel refreshed and alert on 6.5 hours of sleep—an hour less a night than I used to seek. The extra 7 hours a week of usable time that I've been able to add to my schedule have been a true WOW! to me in terms of the incredible amount of "stuff" I've been able to achieve in the extra time.

> Take a "walking meeting" with an associate instead of having a business lunch.

Exercise. You wouldn't think PTs and PTAs would need a reminder about the value of exercise, but the fact is that we all lead busy lives and exercise often gets put on the back burner. There are plenty of ways, however, that you can bring exercise back into your daily routine without it taking a lot of time. Here are a few suggestions:

- If feasible, park a 10-minute walk away from work and walk to and from your car each day.
- Bike to work or church at least once a week.
- Take a "walking meeting" with an associate instead of having a business lunch. (You may be amazed at the effectiveness of this form of communication!)
- Sneak in a short walk before sitting down to lunch. Not only will it feel great, but it may curb your appetite a little and help you keep diet resolutions.

Step Three: Implement "Nows and WOWs!"

As you start off your day, try thinking of your "to-do" list as a list of possibilities rather than tasks. Then take 2 minutes to identify all the "WOWs!" on the list—things you enjoy and that energize you. These may include seeing patients, participating in a special project or putting together an inservice. The next step is to identify all the "Nows"—things you need to do immediately but aren't particularly excited about, like catching up on discharge notes or completing your expense report.

There will be some items on your list that are neither WOWs! nor Nows. Either move them to a later date (where they might become Nows) or delete them if they're neither enjoyable nor essential and are just taking up space on your list of possibilities. That leaves you with only the Nows and WOWs! Next, commit yourself to getting the Nows done before you start the WOWs! This is a key step, since most people jump into the things they enjoy first, when they're full of energy, leaving the less appealing items for later. Committing to knocking out the Nows first will make you complete them more quickly, and you'll get a second shot of energy later in the day as you jump into the things you love doing.

Taking just a few minutes each day to strategize in this way will pay magnificent dividends over the long haul, as you'll be far more productive and energized, and you won't be left dragging your way through unpleasant Nows at the end of the day.

Step Four: Stay in the Game

No matter how cleanly you've lived your life, it's important always to guard against giving in to negative temptations that can drag down your WOW! factor. We face such temptations every day; they range from relatively minor offenses like taking home envelopes and other supplies that are meant for office use to bigger transgressions like taking credit for someone else's work.

The National Basketball Association has an interesting rule—no matter how well you're playing, whatever your overall impact on the game or your team's play, once you receive your sixth foul, you're out of the game. No exceptions, no questions asked. It's the same way in life; moral and ethical lapses add up. Whether or not the referee ever blows the whistle on you and you get caught in these "fouls," they drain the WOW! from you and hold you back from reaching your potential.

Keep this quote from Frank Outlaw in mind the next time you're tempted to commit a foul: "Watch your thoughts; they become words. Watch your words; they become actions. Watch your actions; they become habits. Watch your habits; they become character. Watch your character; it becomes your destiny."[3]

Step Five: Choose WOW!

What was the first impression you gave *yourself* when you woke up this morning? Was it something along the lines of, "Ugh, is that the alarm already?" Or did you immediately remind yourself of all the opportunities you were going to have today to make a difference in someone else's life? Your answer to that question tells me a great deal about how your day actually turned out. The first impressions you give yourself are every bit as important as those you give others.

> Do you want to have a great day? Okay, then—do it!

Do you want to have a great day? Okay, then—do it! Seriously, decide to have a great day and you will! I know, you're thinking, "He doesn't know my boss" or "He doesn't have to live with my teenage son." Excuse me—you're telling me you've given over your power to have a great day to your boss or your son or someone else? Why?

Don't get me wrong. I didn't say anything about your day being perfect. There will be plenty of unexpected events, uncertainties, and unfortunate occurrences—expect them. But don't allow those things to keep you from having a great day. Instead, when those problems and challenges come up, ask yourself these questions from personal development expert Tony Robbins's audiotape series, *Personal Power II*:[4]

1. What could be great about this?
2. What's not perfect yet?
3. What am I willing to do to make it the way I want it?
4. What am I willing to no longer do to make things the way I want them to be?
5. How can I do what's necessary to get the job done and enjoy the process?

I've kept those questions in my wallet for the past several months as reminders to focus on the WOW! Questions 3 and 4, in particular, always put my perspective back on track. If my answer to them is "nothing," then I'd better stop complaining!

Optimistic. Eager. Revitalized. Recharged. Proactive. Ambitious. Positive. Passionate. Visionary. Great. Purposeful. Enthusiastic. Dynamic. Invigorated. Vivacious. WOW! Do these words describe you? You can fill your brain with WOW! or settle for the uninspired "just a job" approach. It's your choice. As for me, make mine WOW!

References

1. Carper J. EatSmart. *USA Weekend*. June 23, 2000;A4.
2. National Sleep Foundation. *ABCs of ZZZZ—When you can't sleep*. Available at www.sleepfoundation.org/sleeplibrary/index.php?secid=&id=53. Accessed March 7, 2006.
3. cybernation.com. Available at www.cybernation.com/quotationcenter/quotelist.php?type=s. Accessed March 7, 2006.
4. Robbins T. *Personal Power II* [audiotape]. Niles, Ill: Nightingale-Conant Corporation; 1996.

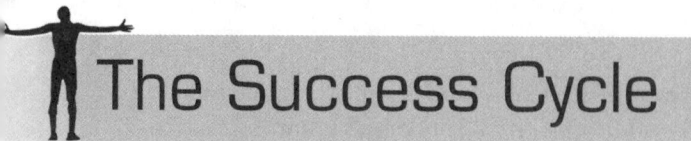

The Success Cycle

This simple tool can help springboard you, your department, and your facility to the next level of performance.

Success for physical therapists (PTs) and physical therapist assistants (PTAs) lies in the positive results we help our patients/clients achieve. In order for any physical therapy practice to survive, however, success also must include bottom-line, dollars-and-cents results.

In short, "no margin, no mission." Without a profit margin, it becomes virtually impossible for us to pursue the mission we've set out to accomplish. We saw this during the dot-com debacle of the late 1990s, as hundreds of companies were highlighted in magazine after magazine for their impressive "employee-friendly" work atmospheres. Company executives spoke of the role that pampering their staffs with incredible perks, such as pool tables and concierge services, played in advancing their missions.

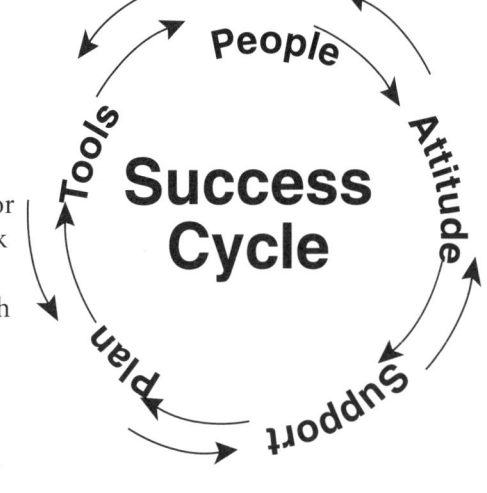

Success Cycle — People, Attitude, Support, Plan, Tools

But where did those companies and those perks end up? When the profit margins disappeared, so, too, did the companies and their missions.

I think it's important to recall the words of Albert Einstein, who said, "Any intelligent fool can make things bigger and more complex. It takes a touch of genius ... to move in the opposite direction." I don't claim to be a genius, but I agree with Einstein that simplicity is key. In keeping with that conviction, I've devised a simple tool that I believe can be extremely helpful in turning around a struggling physical therapy department, or even an entire facility. I call it the Success Cycle.

The Success Cycle essentially is a map to the turnaround process. By separately analyzing each of the following interdependent elements of the cycle, you are likely to discover where—or if—you need to change the way you're doing things.

People

If you've got the wrong people in place, the game's over before it's begun! This process must begin with the leaders. Over the years, I've repeatedly witnessed facilities that have changed their character—and their results—for the better almost overnight as a consequence of new leaders who ushered in new energy and new direction.

But leadership is only the beginning of the quest to get the right people in place. As a Colorado native, I've watched the NBA's Denver Nuggets wade their way through mediocrity for more than a decade. They've tried new plans, new coaches, and new management structures, but the fact is, they can't seem to get the right people together at the right time. A short list of the players who have come and gone reads like a virtual All-Star team—Dikembe Mutombo, Mark Jackson, Nick Van Exel, Jalen Rose, Bobby Jackson. But individuals don't succeed in a vacuum;

the lack of an able supporting cast for each of these superstars has resulted in a decade of failure.

Health care facilities aren't all that different from the Nuggets in this arena. Superstars can fail where teams succeed. The supporting cast is critical to the turnaround and long-term success of any organization. So Phase 1 of the Success Cycle is to look at the people you have in place and determine whether they are getting the chance to be themselves and to really show you what they can do. (There's more on that subject in "Review Your Performance Reviews!" on page 18).

Attitude

You've heard the expression "Attitude is everything"? Well, it may not be everything, but it sure has a massive impact on results. As a national speaker and consultant, I have a chance to see a wide variety of physical therapy teams and facilities around the country. It's not unusual for me to walk through a facility before people arrive in the morning and marvel at the equipment, design, and location, only to become disappointed when the staff gets in and their attitudes paint a less-flattering portrait of the place.

My mom creates magic with the quilts she builds. That magic comes with a cost of time and—of course—materials. Just last week, she told me that she went into a fabric store, but, after spending 5 minutes watching two employees treat each other with disrespect, she left and headed across town to one of the store's competitors. If that was how the first store's staff interacted with one another, she reasoned, how well could she and other customers expect to be treated over the long haul?

If that test is valid for quilting supplies, you can bet it's valid for a physical therapy department. What's the tone of your department? As I note in "Service Matters!" (page 14) mental posturing plays a critical role in customer service, for both internal and external customers.

Support

Even great people with amazing attitudes won't get far if they don't have support from the top. For many supervisors, this means standing back and letting staff do what they do best. For others, it means stepping in and giving staff additional guidance. Often, it simply means listening. What it *doesn't* mean is taking a "my way or the highway" approach.

I'm blessed to have three kids, but each of them learns in quite a different way. When my oldest daughter was learning to ride her bike, she wanted to think about it, get a hug from me, talk about it, get another hug, think about it some more, try it with me holding on to her, and then maybe—possibly—have me run alongside her (after one more hug).

At the other end of the spectrum, her little sister simply wanted to jump on the bicycle and go for it. How effective would it have been for me to have said to her, "No, honey, I want you to think about it for a while, then I'll give you a hug, then ..." simply because that's how I'd done it with her sister?

Managers and leaders must tune into the fact that there are many, many different ways of going about a task. They should make a habit of saying, "I don't know—what do you think would be the best way to go about it?" Being available and supportive doesn't mean looking over the staff member's shoulder—unless the staff member requests that kind of hands-on assistance. For many people, being so closely supervised dries up the creative juices and disengages them from the project.

Plan

Ah, yes, the plan. Where are you headed, and does everyone know it? Do they understand the plan? Did they have an opportunity to help develop it?

Each year my family heads out on vacation. The quickest way for us to get started would be to simply pile the kids in the van and hit the road, without any sort of itinerary. But about 10 minutes down the road, we'd look at each other and wonder if we were headed in the right direction. That's not the most effective way to reach one's destination.

Unfortunately, this often is how businesses go about their daily pursuits—they just jump in the car and go. Where? Oftentimes nowhere. Or the "wrongwhere"!

Whether you are involved with a special program or are running a facility, take the time to sit down with others who are involved and discuss where you're heading. The important thing is not necessarily to spend hours and hours putting together the "perfect" plan. It is valuable, however, to at least take care of the basics: Who will be the program's champions? Where will time and money be invested? What goals are in place for the first month, the first quarter, the first year? Who will provide ancillary support? What type of marketing will be involved?

There's a reason the "no-huddle" offense works only in short bursts in the National Football League. Long-term success requires detailed planning (or at least planning!).

Tools

The remaining piece of the Success Cycle is tools. Marcus Buckingham, in *First, Break All the Rules*,[1] writes that asking the question, "Do I have the materials and equipment I need to do my work right?" is critical to having a motivated and successful team. This doesn't mean that your materials and equipment necessarily must be the best of the best. It means, rather, that the tools needed to get the job done are available.

As I speak around the country on innovation, I'm amazed at the two extremes that exist in this realm. On one end is the manager who won't spend a penny but wants the team to pull together new and exciting programs that will make thousands of dollars for the organization. On the other end is the team member who wants to break the bank on equipment before ever proving that the program is viable.

Both options lead to failure more often than not. The key is to have the necessary tools and to carefully analyze whether an upgrade will provide a reasonable return on investment. I write this column every other month, for example, on a laptop computer. It's not the latest and greatest laptop, but it gets the job done quite nicely. And I sincerely doubt that anyone who reads this column and is considering hiring me as a speaker or consultant cares whether I have the hottest, most cutting-edge computer, as long I can provide the skills and expertise that his or her organization needs. That person isn't about to say, "We can't hire him—his computer is 18 months old." The value of my upgrading to a new computer isn't, at this point, worth the return.

There's no magic pill to success in business—although in glancing at the claims made by the latest business books and magazines, you might be convinced otherwise! If, however, you use the Success Cycle as a guide to analyze your current situation and where you're headed, there's no doubt in my mind that you'll have a better chance of accomplishing your goals.

References
1. Buckingham M, Coffman C. *First, Break All the Rules: What the World's Greatest Managers Do Differently*. New York, NY: Simon & Schuster; 1999.

Beat Burnout!

These seven steps will help you keep the flame lit.

Fellow APTA members, how strong is the fire within you? Is it blazing, or barely flickering? As we try to do more and more in our professional and personal lives with less and less time—continuously shrinking our recovery buffer between one challenge and the next—the pressure keeps building and our passion and energy levels steadily wane. The next step? The dreaded "burnout."

In "Where's the Passion?" (see page 44), I share some ideas for bringing the fire back into your professional life. In this follow-up, I'm going to show you that it's never too late to reassess, regroup, and reenergize. The keys to doing so lie in the following seven steps for beating burnout.

1. Don't Jump to Conclusions

You're just generally tired, unmotivated, discouraged. It must be because of your job, right? Not necessarily! Just about everybody has it up to here with his or her professional responsibilities at some point, but most of us spend only roughly 25% of the 168 hours in each week at work. Could the real, dominant source of your burnout lie in some other aspect of your life?

Ask yourself the following questions before you try and convict your workplace without so much as an evidentiary hearing:

- How are your relationships with those closest to you? I can guarantee you that I'm more upbeat and effective in my professional pursuits when the time I spend with my wife and kids is consistent and meaningful.

- Do you have any health issues? When you're recovering from illness or battling a medical condition, you have that much less energy left for all the things you need to do.

- Has your life undergone any major changes recently? If you'll recall from Psychology 101, just about *any* change causes stress—even good changes, such as getting married or snaring a promotion.

The sooner you can identify the main source of your feelings of burnout, the sooner you can either do something about it or try to put things in perspective and adjust your short-term expectations (depending on the cause).

2. Focus on What You *Can* Control

Some of the most discouraged, grumpy people I know focus on things they cannot control—the weather, the state of the stock market, their grown-up children's choices in life, etc. What's the use?

Face it—a large portion of the circumstances surrounding your life is out of your control. There are few things more stressful and burnout-inducing than putting all your energy into things that won't change regardless of your efforts. One thing you *can* control, however, is how and where you concentrate your energy. Most likely you can have some control over at least one or two of the following things:

- ***The time you leave for work.*** Sometimes leaving 5 minutes early will save you 20 minutes of traffic. Find those drive-time windows and use them to your advantage. Whether or not your work schedule is flexible, you surely can find a better (and less maddening) use for that extra time than spending it sitting in traffic—such as working out, writing e-mails, or running errands near your office.

- ***The people with whom you spend your time.*** Face it, unhappy people are exhausting. Stop spending time with those who suck the energy out of you with their constant complaining. Hang out with engaged, motivated people and you're bound to absorb some of their attitude.

- ***What you do with your free time.*** Are you making sure you always build some unstructured recovery time into your schedule? It may be time to revamp your weekly itinerary and just say "no" to a few things.

You may find that having just a few spare minutes each day, completing one after-work errand, or sharing an extra laugh or two with an upbeat friend or co-worker makes a huge difference in transporting you over the daily hump.

3. Be You

If you've determined that your job is indeed your major source of burnout, consider whether your supervisor is tuned in to what makes you unique. I've written about people's different temperaments and the ways that they most harmoniously interact—see "Get in Sync!" and "Appreciate the Differences!" (on pages 112 and 103 respectively). You might want to give those chapters a look. Each of us has different things that drive us, energize us, make us come alive. For some people it's a chance to make a big impact. For others it's the opportunity to research a specific problem. The energy it takes to do something that doesn't allow you to be yourself may be two or three times what's required to tap into your natural abilities and just be you.

If you feel you could be getting much more out of your work, and that your employer could be getting much more out of you, there's no better time than now to sit down and talk with the person or people who can help make it happen.

4. Get Physical

We're *physical* therapists and *physical* therapist assistants—remember? But how many of us are doing the right things for our own physical well-being? Let's start with the basics:

- *Sleep.* Are you getting enough—could it be that part of your burnout is simple weariness? Or, conversely, are you getting more than enough sleep—shaving time that might be better spent getting things done, diminishing your stress, and making you feel less burned out? Everyone's sleep needs are a little different. You might try increasing or decreasing your sleep duration by 15 minutes each night for a week, gauging your energy level, and seeking a personal equilibrium between time gained and energy diminished.

- *Exercise.* As I note in "Awakening the Wow!" (page 55), even just taking a walk at lunchtime can really rejuvenate you. So, are you doing it yet?

- *Nutrients.* Can you imagine world-class athletes competing on a diet of candy bars and fast food? Of course not. They know the impact food has on performance. Maybe you don't have an Olympic trials competition just around the corner, but what you put into your system is certain to have an impact on how you feel.

- *Stimulants.* We're a coffee nation; that's unlikely to change anytime soon. But here's a key question: Is your caffeine intake under your control, or are you under its control? What would happen if you eliminated the caffeine for just one day? Not doable? If that's the case, that may be a sign that you're taking in enough caffeine each day for it to affect the duration and quality of your sleep—which in turn can greatly contribute to feelings of lethargy and burnout.

5. Stretch

Many PTs use stretching in their practice with patients and clients, but what about in your own life? I'm not talking about joining a yoga or Pilates class, although both are good ideas. Rather, I'm talking about battling burnout by stretching yourself literally or figuratively—targeting something that's outside of your standard "range of motion" or comfort zone—and then going for it.

Depending on your interests, any of the following might be worth consideration:

- Run a 5-kilometer race (or, if you're already a runner, consider setting your sights on a marathon),
- Write a book,
- Join a new club,
- Lose 20 pounds,
- Skydive,
- Build an addition onto your home,
- Take a class (even pursue another degree!), and/or,
- Climb a mountain.

Once you've accomplished one or more of the above, you're likely to feel a welcome boost of energy that may carry over into your daily life.

6. Make Sure Your Star Is in Alignment

Several times each year I lead a "Champions Roundtable" in Colorado that's designed to help keep leaders focused within their professions. One of the roundtable's focal points is a discussion of the star depicted in the accompanying diagram.

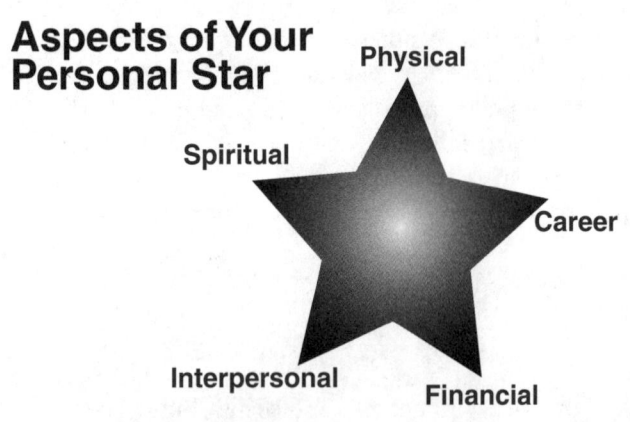

Aspects of Your Personal Star

Physical
Spiritual
Career
Interpersonal
Financial

The star points can be good catalysts for exploring whether your personal star is properly aligned in order for you to experience contentment and fulfillment and avoid burnout. As you look at the star points, what are some of your thoughts? Is there an area you've over- or under-emphasized, perhaps to your overall detriment? Take finances, for example. If you're too focused on this area, it's likely to affect the other points of the star. Maybe your spending habits are contributing to feelings of being behind the economic eight ball, which can contribute to burnout. What if you:

- Purchased a car that was 2 or 3 years old rather than a new one,
- Packed your lunch each day instead of eating out,
- Opted to go without cable television, and/or
- Said "tough beans" to your $4-a-day Starbucks fix?

Don't cut out all the pleasures in your day—that's not balance, and it'll only make you feel more burned out! But if expenditures that you could fairly easily avoid are forcing your star out of alignment, maybe they're worth re-considering. And it won't be just money you're saving—some of these choices (such as cooling off your romance with the TV remote) may benefit the other star points—relieving stress and making you feel better about your life.

7. Do Things Write

A final step toward invigorating your life and fighting burnout is to write out a "to-do" list. Even if you get tired merely *thinking* about all the things that are crowding your itinerary, they seldom look quite so overwhelming when you put them down on paper. And then there's that little rush you'll get when you've completed a task and literally can cross it off the list.

As PTs and PTAs, we play an important role in the lives of so many people. We need to be energized and on top of our game for our patients and clients, and our co-workers, families, and friends depend on us to avoid burnout, too. When the fire within us dims and the candle burns out, the damage can extend far beyond just us.

By the same token, however, a PT or PTA with passion for life can make such a positive impact—in addition to being a much happier and healthier individual. So take the time today to consider your susceptibility to burnout and whether the seven steps outlined here can help you. The new year is no longer so new. It may be time for you to stop resolving to change and actually do something about it. If you try it, you may find that your life will never be the same.

How's That?

In professional planning and in life, it's not so much what you're doing as it is how you're doing it.

Your parents probably started wondering about it before you were born. It's an undercurrent of instruction from your middle school years on. In fact, you'll probably ponder it to some degree throughout your earning life—whatever you end up doing and whatever your level of "success," however you choose to define the word.

What is "it"? That's exactly what "it" is—the "what." The question of *what* you are to do with your life. *What* pursuit best matches your interests, aptitude, and talents? *What* is it that you're best suited to do? *What* will make you happiest and most fulfilled?

We've all met people who seem to have the answer—people who focus from a young age on a certain career, perhaps even a very specific job within that field, and attain their goal and seemingly flourish. But rest assured, even those people sometimes reflect on whether they're doing what they should be doing with their lives. It's human nature to question one's choices and the use of one's potential.

The "what" question is a big motivator of many of the physical therapists (PTs) who attend my Champions Roundtable leadership retreat or seek my personal career-coaching services. Some of them have been working in the profession for more than 20 years, yet the question still lingers: "Am I doing what I'm meant to do?" By that I *don't* mean, as a rule, that they second-guess their decisions to become PTs, but rather that they retain some nagging feeling, however small it may be in some cases, that there are things they should be doing within the profession that they aren't doing.

Ask Not What ...

In working with these PTs, I've come to the conclusion that they're asking the wrong question. Rather than focusing on the "what" in professional-related decision-making, they should be asking themselves "*how*."

Life is in a constant in a state of flux. Look around: Jobs change, companies change, industries change! As a result, that perfect "what"—the dream job that represents exactly what you should be doing with your life—is a moving target. The PT student, for example, spends 2 months in a clinical affiliation at an inpatient rehab facility. He or she has a supportive supervisor, the workplace is mission-driven, co-workers are friendly and professional, and the patients truly appreciate the care they receive. Thinking he or she has found the perfect "what," upon graduation that student pursues an inpatient position advertised in *PT Bulletin Online*. He or she moves into a new home, gets settled in, and gets to work, certain that everything's going to be just great.

But 9 months later, things change. An insurance contract is renegotiated that results in two employees being laid off and tight budgets all around. Staff morale plummets, and that same new graduate finds him- or herself questioning why in the world he or she ever thought this was the perfect practice setting. So the new grad starts to look around and eventually takes a position with an outpatient clinic across town.

Just as before, the honeymoon is good. For the first few months the recent grad is convinced that he or she has made the perfect choice. The euphoria doesn't last long, however. A lack of direction from the recent grad's supervisor sends the young PT into the job-search mode yet again.

This pattern repeats itself countless times around the country, as PT after PT looks fruitlessly for the perfect answer to the question, "What should I be doing with my education, training, and skills?"

The problem is, no individual can control the "what," which is dependent on decisions by and actions of co-workers, patients, supervisors, insurance companies, and government officials.

Change the Question

But the "how"—*how* you perform your job, *how* you deal with the challenges you face—is something upon which you can make an impact, moment by moment, day by day. That's true in professional decision-making and across the board in life.

Viktor Frankl, in his classic book *Man's Search for Meaning*,[1] described the horrors he experienced in Nazi concentration camps and the mental and physical anguish that permeated that existence. He noted that when prisoners focused on the "what"—What was going to happen next? What could possibly stop the Nazis?—there truly was no hope, because the prisoners had no control over those matters. Only those who focused in on what they *could* control—how to make it through each individual day—could stave off utter despair and go on.

On a less-dramatic scale, take the NASDAQ stock drop of 2002-2003. Many people watched the value of their investments rise 30%, 50%, even 85% in a single year in the late 1990s only to watch those gains later disappear and even turn into losses. It was a powerful reminder that the focus must be on the "how" of prudent investing (dollar cost-averaging, investing for the long haul as part of a balanced portfolio, and so on), rather than the "what" of blindly pursuing an ever-changing profit goal.

How Now

The question is, how do you get past the "what," to the "how?" It's not easy, but the following steps will help start you down the path.

- **Identify the "what."** The first step is to pull out your journal or a notebook and begin writing. Start with all your professional responsibilities and priorities—*what* it is you do, and need to do. Next, identify the goals you're pursuing—*what* is it that you want to do? Select the four to six goals that will have the greatest impact on your profession and your life.

- **Identify the "how."** Now it's time to look at your "what" lists—what you're doing now and what you hope to achieve—and think about *how* you go about doing those things, or *how* you plan to get them done. For example, a PT might write down "insurance verification" as one of her responsibilities; it's something she must do if she wants to get paid for her services. Where she has options, however, is in her approach. Does she approach this duty grumpily or amiably, haphazardly or in an organized matter? Similarly, if what she wants to do is open her own practice, how is she pursuing that dream? Actively or passively? By asking questions and researching every aspect of practice ownership, or by waiting until her schedule "settles down a little" to begin those efforts? How that PT lives out each "what" is very much in her control.

> There's only a one-letter difference between saying you've "got" to do something and you "get" to do something.

- **Change one letter.** During a recent Champions Roundtable, we talked a lot about "e-life." You see, there's only a one-letter difference between saying you've "got" to do something (you must do it) and you "get" to do something (you're savoring the opportunity to do it right). But the "e-life" approach makes a big difference in terms of attitude—and often results. Let me illustrate with an example from my own household. Cleaning the house has to rank at or near the bottom of my and our three children's list of fun activities. Two of our favorite things to do, however, are dance around to loud music and surprise mom with something that'll make her smile. So sometimes, while my wife Suzanna is out running errands, the kids and I crank up the dance tunes and "shake it" while we scurry around cleaning as many rooms as we can while she's gone. By living the e-life in Suzanna's absence, we make a tedious task fun, the time flies by, and mommy comes home to a special treat from a loving (if exhausted!) family.

There You Are

What would have happened to the hypothetical new graduate I referenced earlier had she focused on the "how" rather than the "what"? When changing circumstances dimmed the glow of her initial dream job (the "what" she had been pursuing), she could have stepped back and tried to determine how she was responding to the challenges she faced and how well the job was meeting—or potentially could meet—her needs. For example, was she connecting with individual patients and her co-workers? Was she being attentive to her personal fitness? Was she meeting her goal of committing 10% of her salary to savings and another 10% to charity? Was she having a positive impact on the lives of her patients and co-workers? Was she expanding her knowledge base?

That renegotiated insurance contract that upset the new graduate's apple cart might have shifted her strategies for addressing those "how"s, but it certainly didn't eliminate the opportunity to fulfill them. So okay, maybe the changes would've meant tighter schedules and few opportunities to visit with co-workers over coffee. As a result, maybe the PT would have needed to invite colleagues over for dinner or organize a potluck lunch at the office. The potential for connecting with co-workers wasn't eliminated.

Similarly, raises and/or benefits might have shrunk because of tighter finances, but was jumping ship the PT's best option? Perhaps not. Rather than starting over at a different facility, could the PT have approached her supervisor and sought creative ways to regain income and benefits in both the short and long terms?

Money for professional development might not flow so readily within a tight budget, but what other options were available to the PT? Might she have volunteered to teach a course in exchange for a discount on taking another?

The point is, if that PT were focused on the "how" instead of the "what," she might still be at her original practice and enjoying the results. Are there exceptions? Absolutely. But as my mom used to say with regard to marriage, "When you trade partners you don't get rid of problems, you just exchange one set of problems for another." That's pretty good professional advice as well.

I'm writing this piece while returning from the first kid-free vacation with my wife in 8 years—a 3-day trip to the beach. Am I looking forward to leaving that behind, putting on the tie and the dress shoes, and returning to those intense, 12-hour days at the office? Not exactly. But neither am I depressed about it. Why not? Because my life back in the "real world" is darn good: three amazing kids, plenty of food to eat, a warm house in which to live, a loving wife, and many friends. Our "how" is to learn, to love, to leave a legacy of caring. And that "how," frankly, can be more easily fulfilled at the office than it can lying in a hammock with a cool drink in one's hand.

Country music's Clint Black really nailed it when he sang, "Wherever you go, there you are." As you go through your professional and personal life, focus on your "how" and the "what" likely will take care of itself.

Reference
1. Frankl VE. Man's Search for Meaning. Boston, Mass: Beacon Press; 2000.

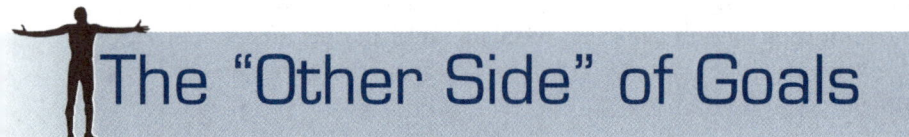

The "Other Side" of Goals

Consider these strategies for better goal attainment—for patients and yourself.

Physical therapists (PTs) know that goals for patients and clients must be specific, measurable, and documented, and that we must review them with the patient or client.[1] It's a meticulous and vital process. Still, in many cases goal attainment proves elusive. There are many reasons for that, of course, but I see some basic things we can do better to help increase success levels.

Look around your city or town—what do you see? A ton of overweight people, right? (All right, several tons!) Now ask yourself, how many of your patients or clients would have less need for physical therapy—or perhaps no need for it at all—if they were at or near their ideal weight? The fact, however, is that every day in this country, countless numbers of people pledge to lose 10 pounds—and countless numbers of people are in the process of failing to do so. Why should we think many of these same people will be able to meet their physical therapy goals?

This is where what I call the "other side" of goals comes in. If you'll try the strategies I'm about to suggest, I believe you can enhance the likelihood that your patients—and you yourself—will be more successful in consistently achieving goals, in physical therapy and in life.

Success in Support

How'd your day go today? I'm going to make an educated guess that your answer has a lot to do with how your front office team member's day went. I'm right, aren't I? If you have a good relationship with your front office team member and he or she had a good day, you probably did too. And the same can work in reverse. That kind of mutual support is a critical to the success of any clinic or facility.

Support comes in various forms. It may be a case of someone saying just the right word or phrase when you feel as if you're ready to throw in the towel. At the Triathlon World Championships in New Zealand in December 2003, a spectator's words may have helped cut a couple minutes off my time. Rather than shouting the usual "You look great!" (yeah, right!), he calmly said, "Looking smooth, excellent form, you're almost gliding." Whether or not that really was true, it reminded me how I should look, and made me redouble my efforts to stay in form. I was on a multiple-loop course and started looking forward to going by that guy again and again—someone I'd never seen before and almost surely never will see again.

Does your patient or client have anyone besides you in her life who will ask if she's doing her exercises, keeping her posture, changing her lifting motion as instructed? Who's on your patient's "team," as it were? Ask! Make it a high priority, when you're sitting down with a patient or client, to identify a person or people he can ask to push and motivate him, just like that guy in New Zealand motivated me. With the help of a support team—even a "team" of just one individual—the patient's or client's chances for goal attainment can escalate considerably.

Keep It Positive

My wife and I have three kids. The youngest, Josh, is 5 at this writing. If he's walking down the stairs with a glass of milk and I say to him "Don't spill your milk!" what have I done to the chances he'll spill it? I've increased them, by putting the thought in his head and introducing a negative goal.

I'd like to write a weight-loss book titled *It's Not About The Weight!* (Apologies to Lance Armstrong, who wrote *It's Not About the Bike*.) If people would stop focusing on losing weight and instead focus on pursuing fitness, they'd improve their chances for success. I mean, if you're driving a car, don't you focus on where you're going, rather than on where you're not going? You generally say "Turn here," right?—not, "Don't turn there." In relationship terms, does a husband strengthen his marriage by making it his primary goal not to have an affair? Ridiculous! His aiming to be a good spouse and do everything he can to keep lines of communication open will serve the union a lot better. Yet, too often, we focus on telling people what not to do, rather than giving them positive goals.

Have you fallen into that pattern with your patients? It's my feeling that instructions such as "Don't lift with your legs straight" or "Don't lean over at your desk" are less likely to motivate patients to comply than telling them what it is you do want them to do. Turn those instructions around: "It's best to lift this way and sit at your desk that way. You'll be glad you did." Encourage patients, don't discourage them.

A Journey of Recovery

> I've read of managers who've locked office doors and shut down computer networks just to force employees to, well, get a life.

The majority of orthopedic patients benefit from interspersing within the home program occasional lighter-intensity, or "recovery" days. In an optimal scenario, the patient visits the PT perhaps 2 or 3 days a week and follows the PT's home exercise instructions on the days between physical therapy sessions. But in these days of higher co-pays and less-frequent visits to the PT, the PT may only see the patient once a week. When that's the case, are you paying sufficient attention to varying the intensity of the home program on a day-by-day basis—with an eye toward not only ensuring sufficient recovery time, but also toward battling patient boredom and its byproduct, noncompliance?

The "other side" of goals here is making sure the patient knows why varied intensity level within, and strict adherence to, the home program is so very important. The PT who does that, while taking care to break up the monotony, has a much better chance of securing patient compliance than the PT who doesn't.

Patient goals aside for a moment, in your personal goals, are you building in time to "recover," or are you moving from one goal to the next, speeding toward a date with burnout? If you're a manager, are you giving your staff a chance to recover on weeknights and weekends, or are you overworking them month after month? Tough times may require digging deep and going the extra mile for a limited time, but doing so on a regular basis is a formula for disaster—on both the personal-performance and the employee-turnover fronts.

I've read of managers who've locked office doors and shut down computer networks just to force employees to, well, get a life. Not only is constant overwork bad for body and soul, but active and joyful pursuit of a hobby at home during those extra hours actually can energize an employee, making him or her a better and more productive worker in your clinic or facility.

Make It Rewarding

One final note about goals: Don't forget the rewards. Laud your patients as they achieve each goal. They may not see the progress you do. Point it out to them, and celebrate it!

On a personal level, the same holds true. Rewards big or small—an expensive toy or a dinner out—can keep you moving forward when your energy wanes. Tie rewards to specific accomplishments, and be sure to "pay up" when you achieve the target. You earned it!

Reference
1. *Guide to Physical Therapist Practice.* Revised 2nd Ed. Alexandria, Va: American Physical Therapy Association; 2003.

Look Beneath the Surface

If all you see ahead of you are clear skies and open water, maybe it's time to dive under and survey your professional and personal life from a different perspective.

As each of us made our way through our physical therapist (PT) or physical therapist assistant (PTA) studies, we received plenty of feedback on our performance. Tests, homework assignments, practical exams—they all took the pulse of how well we were doing at our "job" of being students. Upon graduation, many of us were only too happy to leave all of that behind us. No more people looking over our shoulder and instructing, guiding, and grading us. Finally, the freedom to treat patients without those pressures!

But wait a minute. How do we really know, as gainfully employed PTs and PTAs, how we're doing? Maybe we've had a recent performance review. Perhaps our organization has conducted a customer satisfaction survey that indicates how well we're connecting with patients and meeting their needs. We attend professional development and continuing education classes that offer us windows into what we do and don't know, and perhaps how we stack up compared with our classmates. But what kinds of performance assessments are we getting all the other days of the year?

Caught on Video

Feedback—from someone who knows what he or she is talking about—is vital to our growth and improvement. I was reminded of this (rather, I was embarrassed to be reminded) on a recent Saturday, when my daughter Ashley and I attended a swimming workshop together.

(A little background: Three years ago I couldn't swim a lick. But midnight madness overtook me; I signed up very late one night to compete in the Escape

Section 3 — It's Your Attitude   77

from Alcatraz Triathlon—effectively forcing myself to learn to swim, or possibly die trying! Since that time I've worked hard on my swimming, and I've seen some decent improvement.)

I was in my daddy mode when I accompanied Ashley to the swimming workshop. I saw it as a chance for us to spend some time together and for her to gain some valuable knowledge. I wasn't really there to learn anything myself—not after all the reading and practicing I'd done over the past 3 years to get where I was with my swimming technique.

Underwater videotaping captured each of us in action as we swam the length of the pool. I swam faster than many of the other workshop attendees and detected stroke errors in some of the participants that I knew I wasn't making. When we all gathered in the conference room afterward to review with the coach what we'd looked like in water, I assumed he'd find very little to critique in my performance, but that Ashley would get some good feedback on how to improve her form.

I would be absolutely wrong in my self-assessment, however. The experience was not pleasant. While I looked fine above the water, the underwater video footage revealed—and the coach pointed out—my too-short stroke, limited pull-through, quick exit, and minimal rotation. In fact, he had little good to say about my performance.

At first, I felt utterly deflated. I'd been putting a lot of time into improving my stroke, typically getting up at 4:30 am several days a week to swim with a local masters team. And this was the result? But my next reaction to the critique was considerably more constructive. On second thought, I reasoned, this actually was awesome news! (Okay, so maybe I am, on balance, more of a glass-half-full kind of guy.) When I got to thinking about it, I looked at it like this: I'd been able in the previous year to trim a significant amount off my 1500-meter open water time, but the video was telling me I still had room for improvement. Outstanding!

What I realized was that the most discouraging thing that could've happened to me at that workshop would've been if I'd been told that I'd more or less reached my peak, and that there was no realistic way I'd ever get any faster. Instead, upon close—and, yes, painful—examination by an expert, I'd been handed a blueprint for improvement.

Underwater Cameras

Now, let me ask you: How much feedback have you sought in the following areas of your life?

- *Clinical skills.* You're dedicated, and you feel as if you're pretty much on top of your clinical game. And maybe you are. But is "pretty much" good enough?

- *Management.* You note that everyone says you're a great manager. Again, maybe you are. But what do you expect your employees to say—that the boss isn't "all that"? Have you asked any of your superiors for a truly honest, constructive assessment of your management abilities and style?

- *Relationships.* You say that things are great in your marriage, with your kids, with your co-workers and friends. True? There's nothing you could do to better nurture those relationships?

- *Finances.* You joke that you have "the best life credit can buy." That's funny! But is it at least a little bit true? If so, the joke may be on you, and you may need to do something about it.

- *Health.* Just because the word "physical" is in your occupational description doesn't mean you're in the kind of shape you should be in. Speaking of physicals, when's the last time you had one?

Are you willing to swallow hard and try to determine how you're really doing in each area? Do you sincerely want to know? The feedback you receive could change your professional, and perhaps your personal, life. Here are some moves you may want to consider if you're serious about taking "underwater snapshots" of yourself:

- *Clinical skills.* Have you considered putting your skills to the test by joining a study group and seeking specialist certification through APTA? Are you willing to visit www.apta.org and search the American Board of Physical Therapy Specialties' online directory of certified clinical specialists for an individual who can help you reach the professional goal that he or she already has achieved? How about testing and strengthening your clinical skills by seeking an APTA-credentialed postprofessional clinical residency or fellowship?

- *Management.* Have you sat down with your supervisor and asked him or her to pinpoint at least one thing you could be doing better—and to hold you accountable for improving? (If your manager tries to tell you you're doing everything well, respectfully suggest that he or she is insane! Because nobody does everything well, and you really want to grow.) Have you looked around for a mentor—someone at your management level who seems truly to "get it," or someone at the next-higher level who's willing to ask you some tough questions and offer his or her "underwater" feedback? Have you visited the Members Mentoring Members site at www.apta.org?

- *Relationships.* Have you considered participating in a marriage or family retreat, and/or soliciting honest feedback from people who've seen you "in action" to help you better see where you could stand to work a little (or maybe a lot) harder in your relationships with family members, friends, and co-workers? To quote that line from the movie *A Few Good Men*, can you handle the truth? My wife will ask me, "Do you want real feedback, or just agreement?" I need to put a lot of thought into which option I choose!

- **Finances.** Have you read *The Richest Man in Babylon?*[1] It stuffs a lot of sage, age-old advice into a small package. Consider enlisting a friend to read it, too, and then compare notes with him or her. Don't share your private financial numbers, but be honest about how you're doing financially. If you can save and invest at least 10% of your income, give another 10% to worthy causes, and live on the rest, it's likely that your financial picture will be sound in the long run. A simple thing like accountability can turn a nice "book idea" into practical reality.

- **Health.** Model it to your patients—don't merely lecture it. I recently got my cholesterol tested for the first time. High cholesterol can be a silent killer, even for people who are in good shape. Have you taken the time to get your baseline reading? How about determining your body fat percentage? Get a thorough medical checkup. If you don't belong to a gym or health club, what better time than now to get signed up? Don't hesitate to consult experts who can assess how you look beneath the surface.

Yes, it's great to be through with the pressures of school, but we're cheating ourselves, our patients, our families, our friends, and our colleagues if we graduate ourselves from making sure we're doing everything we can to measure up at work and in life. So don't simply rely on your perceptions of yourself. Be willing to take that look underwater to see how you're really doing.

Reference
1. Clason G. *The Richest Man in Babylon*. New York, NY: Bantam Books; 1989 (reissue).

Sport as Life

Tendencies of an All-Star

Become an all-star in your profession.

Let's go back to 1990. For Denver Broncos fans, there was little hope for the future. Their team had just gone 5-11, in spite of a talented quarterback by the name of John Elway and several veteran players. However, things can change quickly, and that change often comes from unexpected places. Shortly after this mediocre season, a relatively unknown player by the name of Terrell Davis joined the team as the 196th player and the 21st running back chosen in the draft. Soon after, the Broncos went on to win back-to-back Super Bowls, while this "unknown" player became the fourth running back in history to run for 2,000 yards in a single season.

Just as in professional sports, our field is loaded with talent. But talent alone isn't enough anymore. To be an all-star, you have to possess certain tendencies that affect the entire team. Let's look at the characteristics of an all-star and how you can become one in your profession.

The Big Picture

True all-stars understand the importance of all roles, not just one. It's difficult to enhance the value of those around you when you're focused only on a single role. Ice hockey hall-of-famer Wayne Gretzky demonstrated this understanding of the big picture. Take note of how *Sports Illustrated*[2] described him following his retirement:

It's difficult to overstate Gretzky's impact on the game. He is both hockey's greatest scorer and its greatest ambassador...he leaves the game with a mind-numbing 61 NHL records, many of which will never be broken. He averaged 203 points/year over a 6-year period—No other NHL player has ever scored even 200 points. With all that said, Gretzky himself says, "Ten years from now, they won't even talk about my goal scoring; it'll just be my passing."

So what does that mean for PTs? It means we all need to understand the big picture of the business we're in, including the key indicators that drive our business. Does anyone still believe the notion: "If I have great hands, nothing else matters"? If so, it's time for those people to expand their perspective. You cannot succeed without strong clinical skills, but clinical skills alone no longer are enough.

Entrepreneurialism

Another key to being an all-star is entrepreneurialism. Whether you create a new program or invent a new piece of equipment, become an entrepreneur in your own practice. You can do so in the following ways:

- *Take back what we gave away when there weren't enough PTs.* This includes physical fitness, wellness, and health; Pilates; hand therapy, and respiratory therapy. Nobody is better trained to do these things (among others) than PTs. Let's take them back.

- *Become an "intrapreneur."* The 3M Company, famous for its Post-It Notes®, is known for its creativity and introducing new products. It does this through supporting "intrapreneurs" (entrepreneurs within the company). Do you have a creative idea that falls outside your facility's "standard" programs? Approach your employer with a realistic, self-directed plan, and there's great potential for success. Not only will this enhance your job security, but you'll be working on something you love, every day.

- *Create something brand new on your own.* Fan your personal entrepreneurial fire with something entirely crazy. In *The Circle of Innovation*,[3] Tom Peters quotes the late Hajime Mitarai, a president of Canon: "We should do something when people say it is crazy. If people say something is 'good,' it means someone else is already doing it." Even if the pursuit doesn't work out, it makes you well-rounded and smarter for having tried.

Network

Not only does an entrepreneurial pursuit make you a well-rounded person and employee, it also expands your network—a critical area of growth for any all-star PT wanting to make a difference.

In *Dig Your Well Before You're Thirsty*,[4] Harvey MacKay tells a story of his daughter when she was in college. She was seeking a waitress position at a local restaurant, and the competition for the position was fierce. Her solution? Access her network, of course. She sought support from all of her friends, contacts, and classmates. By the time she went in for the interview, she was able to hand the hiring manager a list of people who had committed to frequenting the restaurant if she were chosen for the position. With his eye on the bottom line, the employer knew that she was the best candidate for the job.

How's your network? It's been said that there are six degrees of separation between you and anyone else in the world, meaning that almost any two people are connected in six steps or less if you follow the right path. How about tracing your path to key employers, physicians, and insurance contacts? Like MacKay's daughter, your connections will have a positive impact on your organization's bottom line through increased referrals and product line growth. And, if you are ever looking for a new position, nothing beats a strong network. A strong network, both inside and outside the workplace, can be the difference between the average and the all-star PT.

Initiative

All-stars don't restrict themselves to the job description or the 40-hour week. While they're aware of the position description, they see it along the lines of a minimum daily requirement. They make certain that the job is covered, but they don't stop there. Rather, all-stars exceed the expectations of the position and can be counted on to be at their best, day in and day out, usually in a way that benefits not just themselves but also their co-workers or the larger group around them.

Take Cal Ripken Jr, for example. He played 2,632 consecutive baseball games without a day off. That was 16 years of playing every game—not just showing up, but competing at the professional level.

If we want to be all-stars, we can't merely show up. Having initiative means more than just sending a note to your supervisor about a new idea. It means championing an idea that is close to the core of the organization (such as quality, cost, or service) and doing your research about things you know are important to your supervisor, such as time involved, costs, and realistic benefits to the organization.

If you're a student or a job-seeker, this may be demonstrated by finding out which PTs best demonstrate those traits supervisors look for. Approach those PTs about spending a few hours with them to pick up some pointers. Not only are you, then, getting pointers from folks who have the drive, but, better yet, you are expanding your network to include the stars of the organization.

Emotional Bank Account

One of the greatest stories from Denver Broncos lore took place in the AFC Championship game against the Cleveland Browns in 1986. The Broncos needed a touchdown with less than 2 minutes remaining (and at their own 2-yard line), and the situation looked hopeless. As the players gathered in the huddle, with the entire season on the line, one of the Broncos' offensive linemen leaned in and said, with a completely straight face, "Well, we've got 'em right where we want 'em." This ridiculously comical statement loosened the players and reunited them. Was the 98-yard, game-winning drive that followed a direct result of the comment? Probably not, but the player's comment did have a positive impact at a critical time.

What's it like to work with you? An all-star may have an occasional need to push, but not until the "emotional bank account" has a few deposits in it. Think about walking into a bank and asking to withdraw $1,000. The teller's response is based on your deposits up to that point. If you had previously deposited $10,000, then the teller will gladly give you the requested $1,000, thanking you in the process. On the other hand, if you've only deposited $10, you're out of luck.

Your relationships with your coworkers are very similar. If you focus your time on helping others succeed and showing appreciation for those around you, then you've made deposits. If at some point you need to make a withdrawal under pressure, it's okay.

Just as people with a strong network can get things done more quickly because they know the right people, all-stars who excel at interpersonal relationships get better results because people want to help them out. We all have people for whom we give that extra effort and others for whom we do the least possible. Usually that commitment is tied to the deposits that have been made. The more deposits you make, the better the results you get in return.

New Things

> The most successful PTs in the next decade will be the ones with a niche but who aren't confined by that niche.

All-stars, by definition, are at the top of their game. People come to them to learn. But that's no reason for all-stars to stop learning themselves. In fact, the thought never even enters the minds of all-stars. They know that if they are not growing, they are falling behind.

Read without ceasing, and invest in your future by pursuing courses frequently, even if it's out of your own pocket. Choose articles and courses that will make you a "broad-based specialist." Although the term sounds like an oxymoron, I am convinced that the most successful PTs in the next decade will be the ones with a niche (be it wellness, women's health, golf performance, etc) but who aren't confined by that niche. Instead, as generalists, they will be able to fill any gap needing to be filled and, at the same time, develop the niche and bring business to the organization that otherwise would not be there.

And be sure not to stop with the clinical aspects. The other key differentiator over the next decade will be an understanding of the nonclinical aspects, such as marketing, strategic planning, and at least a basic understanding of the "numbers." That doesn't mean you need to rush out to pursue an MBA. Rather, ask questions and read periodicals in addition to *PT*, *Physical Therapy*, and *JOSPT*, such as *Healthcare Executive* or *Modern Healthcare*. A couple of outstanding books that also can give you a head start on the marketing side include *Selling the Invisible* by Harry Beckwith and *Rain Making* by Ford Harding. Your goal isn't to become an expert in these areas; it's to keep from being blindsided.

One of my professors during my days at the Washington University School of Medicine who served as a great example of an all-star who sees learning as an ongoing process, was Shirley Sahrmann, PT, PhD, FAPTA. "You'll get there," she told the class. "Remember, it's not that I'm all that smart. I just try to learn one thing new every day... and I'm really old!"

Communication Skills

Another key differentiator in the next decade will be an ability to communicate effectively, both verbally and in writing. That doesn't necessarily mean speaking publicly or writing articles, although, those are valuable skills to develop as we enter a new age as a profession. The primary issue instead is: Can you get your message across to your audience? The method you choose will depend on that audience.

Consider Sammy Sosa. English is not his first language. But can anyone forget his incredible communication during his homerun surge with Mark McGwire in 1998? His simple way of communicating—kissing his fingers and tapping his heart—got his message across to millions of people all over the globe, and at year's end, he was voted the league's MVP.

Would he have been seen in such a positive light if he'd sat back and said, "I don't yet have a complete grasp of English yet, so I'll play hard but just keep to myself." It's doubtful. Thankfully, we'll never know, because Sosa learned to communicate in a simple, yet incredibly effective way, winning the hearts of millions in the process.

In a similar way, each of us must learn to communicate effectively—with patients, certainly, but also with physicians, case managers, employers, and others to whom we want to express the value of physical therapy. Without this skill, our profession risks being left out.

Attitude

The year was 1997. The Utah Jazz and Chicago Bulls were knotted up at two games apiece in a seven-game series for the NBA Championship. It looked to be Chicago's toughest test to date in its run of championships. This game was likely to set the tone, with the winner taking a huge edge into the remainder of the series.

Leading up the game were reports that Michael Jordan was fighting a stomach virus. He was completely dehydrated, had been unable to keep any food down in the past 24 hours, and was unable to sleep most of the previous night as a result. Bulls fans worldwide had little hope. Without Michael, the Bulls simply were a different team.

But Jordan had different plans. Instead of excusing himself to the bench or locker room as a result of his circumstances, he approached the game with a "yes" attitude.

Clearly on the verge of exhaustion, Michael played a game that no sports fan who witnessed the performance will ever forget. Time after time, he reached down deep into his reserves and found the will to continue. And by continue, I don't mean simply survive or "get by," knowing everyone would excuse a subpar performance due to the illness. Instead, he did the things that only Michael could do, culminating the performance with the game-winning 3-point shot in the closing seconds.

Having given everything he had to the game, he required assistance from his teammates to leave the floor when the final buzzer sounded. When the dust cleared, Michael had finished with 38 points, and his team had emerged victorious and eventually went on to win the series.

In similar situations, you have two choices: You can give up and say, "It's really too bad," or you can dig deep and make things happen, regardless of the circumstances. Attitude really is everything when it comes to being an all-star. For our profession to thrive, we all must bring that "yes" attitude to the table every single day.

The opportunities are there, but it's going to take all-stars to get it done. Pulitzer Prize-winning journalist William Raspberry once said, "People who believe a problem can be solved tend to get busy solving it." I believe. How about you?

References
1. Swift EM. *Sports Illustrated*. April 26, 1999. 35.
2. Peters T. *The Circle of Innovation*. New York, NY: Vintage Books; 1997.
3. MacKay H. *Dig Your Well Before You're Thirsty*. New York, NY: Doubleday; 1997.

'Tri'ed and True Tactics for Professional Success

The triathlon as a learning tool.

I'd long admired triathletes, but I'd never seen myself participating in that kind of test of physical endurance until earlier this year. After all, I'd spent very little time in the pool, my bicycle was 17 years old, and I hadn't run seriously since college. Me, a triathlete? Not a chance!

But then something changed. I started thinking about how, in my speaking engagements to groups of physical therapists (PTs) and other professionals, a recurrent message is that amazing things happen to you when you keep a solid mental posture. Turning my thoughts to the goal of completing a triathlon, it suddenly seemed like the perfect time for me to put what I'd been preaching into practice on a personal, physical level.

The next thing I knew, I was signed up for a half-"Ironman" triathlon, which consists of a 1.2-mile swim, a 56-mile bike ride, and a 13.1-mile run. (More later on why I selected this particularly grueling event as my first triathlon.)

With only 6 weeks in which to train after I'd made my decision, I had a lot of lessons to learn, and fast! The things I discovered while training for and participating in the triathlon, I've since come to realize, are just as applicable to our practices as they are to successfully completing an endurance event.

Phase I: The Coaching

Because I was a triathlon rookie, finding the right coach was particularly critical. As a PT/ATC myself, I knew I would be a tough client to satisfy. I decided to go with a highly respected "virtual" coaching system for endurance athletes (www.trainright.com) that has helped prepare seven-time Tour de France winner Lance Armstrong and many of the world's top triathletes for competition.

I received my coaching online and over the phone. My coach set up a training plan that was specific to me and included such details as establishing my ideal heart rate during each workout. In addition to planning my workouts, he gave me occasional pep talks over the phone. The result was a rapid rise in both my fitness and confidence levels.

Serious athletes wouldn't consider going it alone in their training. So why is it that we think we can go it alone in enriching and advancing professionally? Often it's because we don't realize that many great resources are available to all of us. Consider these professional "coaching" options:

- **Mentors.** Select two or three people who are a step or two ahead of you on the professional ladder or are otherwise in a place where you'd like to be. Ask if you can take them to breakfast or lunch and pick their brains. Most people rarely seek such help, so the individuals you ask will likely feel complimented, and a very valuable relationship may result. In this way I've gained as a mentor Ed Oakley, author of *Enlightened Leadership: Getting to the Heart of Change*, and the time he has spent with me—asking me the tough questions and holding me accountable for my professional-development actions and lack thereof—has been incredibly helpful. But please, be sure to treat your mentors' time like the precious commodity that it is—maximize your face, phone, and e-mail time with these experts by preparing specific questions for them and storing up ideas on which you'd like their "spin."

- **Peers.** Peers can provide a valuable sounding board for your professional aspirations. Form a group of two to six people whose professional goals are similar to yours. Share ideas and strategies and make each other accountable for follow-through. For example, attend a continuing education class as a group and meet afterward to discuss it. Or, if you're pursuing a management track, perhaps meet quarterly with your peer group to discuss a case study from the *Harvard Business Review* or another management-related publication. You may gain a treasure trove of professional information and guidance through your interaction with your peer group.

- **Tapes.** The audiobook industry is expanding rapidly in response to the demands of our busy lives and, in particular, ever-lengthening commutes to and from work. Consider joining a business/professional titles-oriented audiobook club (investigate your options on the Internet and in your local telephone directory), or at least investing a few dollars on a different audiobook each month by one of the nationally known experts on professional enhancement and advancement, such as Tom Peters, Stephen Covey, or Peter Senge.

- **Magazines.** If you're familiar with my columns in *PT—Magazine of Physical Therapy*, you're already receiving a good professional resource as a benefit of your APTA membership. *PT Magazine* offers a variety of feature articles and shorter pieces that contain information and ideas you can use to enhance and advance professionally. But beyond *PT Magazine*, by paying just a few dollars a month, you can stay up-to-date on the latest professional insights from around the globe by subscribing to such magazines as *Inc, Fast Company,* and *Business 2.0.*

Phase II: The Preparation

When people ask me to pinpoint the most difficult aspect of the triathlon, I think most of them expect me to talk about the intervals on the track, or the long swims, or the 3-hour bike rides. But to me, none of those things qualifies as the toughest part.

The most difficult task for me, without a doubt, was getting out of bed in the morning when the rest of the world was sleeping! The training time required to get up to speed (so to speak) in three very demanding physical activities—coupled with the fact that I'm not a professional triathlete and thus don't have sponsors to pay my rent while I do nothing but train—means I had to get started at 4:15 am or earlier on most training days. There were many mornings on which I was extremely tempted to just stay in bed. Hey, what difference would it make if I knocked off for one day, right?

Well, it would've made a big difference! I never acted on those temptations, and I'm glad I didn't. Come race day, I found that the consistency and sense of discipline I'd instilled in myself while training was invaluable.

As PTs, how often do we take the easy road because it's comfortable? How often do we follow the crowd instead of doing what we know we really need to do? Making the demanding choices, even when nobody else is looking, is what makes champions!

Another important part of my triathlon preparation was all the preparatory advice I received. As a rookie triathlete, I had a lot to learn, and the helpful tips came from many directions. One experienced triathlete advised me, for instance, to tie a balloon to my bicycle so that I could find the bike quickly while making the transition—along with 400-plus other participants—from the swimming to the biking segment. "Pick up some aero bars to allow you to stay in lower position" on the bicycle, another savvy veteran suggested. (Aero bars are handle-bar extensions that facilitate aerodynamic riding.) From a third triathlete I received this valuable tip: "Let your bike, not your body, move as you climb hills." (This saves the rider both energy and time.)

Cumulatively, those and other preparatory tips would make a big difference in improving my performance. So ask yourself: In your profession, are you seeking out and paying attention to the views and knowledge of your peers, your employees, your patients/clients, outside experts? Each individual's ideas and suggestions can help move you incrementally forward. Their collective advice may help propel you a long way toward achieving your professional goals.

Just before the race was to start, I told an experienced triathlete that this was not only my first half-Ironman, but also my first triathlon. "You're kidding!" he exclaimed, clearly shocked and a bit pitying. "Why in the world would you do this race as your first triathlon?"

I didn't mention that he was about the 20th person to ask me that question in the past month, and I didn't reveal that one of my prime motivators was the simple fact that most people didn't think I could do it. I just shrugged, wished him luck, put on my wetsuit for the initial swimming segment—and ended up finishing the race about an hour ahead of him.

Who are the doubters and outright naysayers in your professional life? Do you let them bring you down—or do you further build your foundation for professional success by turning their "can't do" spirit into fuel for the fire of your ambition?

Phase III: The Race

> I noticed that I actually felt a surge of energy whenever I encouraged others along the way—including those who were passing me.

The gun sounded, and hundreds of us hit the water—embarking on an adventure that would take most of us 5 to 8 hours to complete. This was the moment at which all of our training and devotion would be tested to the extreme. I was to learn some important lessons during this phase:

- ***Encouragement builds strength.*** During a long event like the half-Ironman, energy aids such as Powerbars® and Accelerade® drinks help, but I found that one of my most powerful energy sources was the encouragement that flew freely among the competitors. Interestingly, I noticed that I actually felt a surge of energy whenever I encouraged others along the way—including those who were passing me.

Does encouragement in your work setting flow freely? Is it a place where people regularly accomplish the seemingly impossible thanks to the support that surrounds them? Are you an active part of this positive atmosphere?

- ***Poorly expressed encouragement can actually sap strength.*** As I neared the end of the run—and thus the triathlon—I ran up to a guy who was struggling and said, "Just one more lap. Let's finish strong together!" It turned out, however, that what I'd meant as encouragement hurt rather than helped because I didn't realize he was nearing the end of only the first of two laps. It served only to remind the exhausted runner that he had an entire lap to go. His spirit seemed to sag even more, right before my eyes.

It's critical in any successful organization to provide people with encouragement, but watch the words you use. If I had it to do over again, I might have said something to the struggling guy like, "Wanna push together?"—

emphasizing the partnership, regardless of a potential difference in our finish targets. In the same way, we all best benefit—and benefit others—professionally by emphasizing and encouraging the attainment of goals. Words count. Be careful how you use them.

- ***One muscle matters more than any other—the heart.*** It can be a little intimidating to look around at the start of a triathlon. The muscles on some of those folks are huge! Physical strength certainly plays a part once the gun sounds, but when it comes down to the final lap, it's all about gutting it out and promising yourself that you will finish—and that's all heart, baby!

Things aren't much different in your clinic, are they? An applicant can come in with an amazing résumé or a huge reputation, but it's the person who pours his or her heart into his or her responsibilities who gets the best results. That isn't to say that solid credentials, and the skills and knowledge you gain while pursuing them, aren't important. But it's your heart—your dedication—that counts the most and will hold you in best stead.

And, speaking of heart, we all know that our profession presents many challenges along with the rewards—particularly in the current and foreseeable health care climate. There are days when each of us finds it difficult to provide the kind of exceptional service to patients/clients for which PTs are known. But persevering at such times and never compromising our devotion to excellence is a form of heart, too.

The Finish? Or Just the Start?

When I crossed that finish line, my feeling of accomplishment was overwhelming. It was definitely a moment I won't ever forget. Very soon after that, however, I felt that the time was ripe for additional challenges. I completed another triathlon 2 weeks later and ran a marathon the following month. There's no such thing as resting on your laurels—there always are new tasks to tackle, new battles to fight!

How about you? Your clinic is running on all cylinders—you just had your best month in recent history and all the doctors are singing your praises. Is it time to relax? Or is it time to pass around the high fives, then set the next goal? Your answer will go a long way toward determining your long-term success. My advice? Keep on "tri"ing!

When the Playing Field Changes

"Tri" these three steps to successful professional advancement.

"Toto, I've a feeling we're not in Kansas anymore."

Those famous words were uttered by Dorothy when she arrived in the land of Oz. Things had changed. The field of play was different. The things she'd always done likely wouldn't be as effective as they once had been.

Do you know how she felt? I certainly do! In December 2003 I competed in the Triathlon World Championships in New Zealand. It was an exciting opportunity, but I quickly learned that the field within which I normally compete had changed—drastically.

The World Championships pit the top 15 amateur triathletes in each age group from each participating country (50 nations were represented in New Zealand) in a competition that consists of a 1500-meter (about 1-mile) swim, a 26-mile bicycle leg, and a 10.2-kilometer (6-mile-plus) run. To get there in the first place, I had to qualify in my gender/age group (males 35-39) in the US. The swim is the weakest of my three events, so in the typical race, I'm used to having to make up significant time on my competition during the bike and the run. Here in the States, that's not a problem. I'll come out of the swim in the middle of the pack and usually catch up with all but a few of my competitors by the end of the race.

But this wasn't a "typical" race by any stretch of the imagination. I swam one of the better races of my first year as a triathlete, but as I came out of the water, I realized there weren't many people behind me anymore. (Okay, honestly, there was almost no one behind me!). But, no problem, right? Well, at the World Championships, it was a problem. I may have had a leg up on most of the competition back home in the bike and the run, but in New Zealand everyone was strong on those elements. And they just happened to be good swimmers too. Ouch!

When all was said and done (ie, swum, biked, and run!), I had moved up, finishing 457th out of 1,320 competitors. But I still felt it was nothing to get too excited about. If I hope to be competitive (which, to me, means being among the top 100 amateur triathletes in the world), that experience taught me that things must change. I can't just do things the same way I've done them against local competition and hope to make a splash on the world scene. I need to make some changes.

As physical therapists (PTs), there are many times when our playing field changes. It happens when we take on a new challenge, step into a new position, or pursue an advanced degree. Whether you're training for a triathlon or striving to better yourself professionally, there's a triumvirate of critical steps you must take to get to the finish line and achieve your goals.

Assess. As a triathlete at the local level, I could get away with having a weakness. When I competed against the best athletes in the world, however, weakness in any area of my game was something I no longer could afford. Since returning home from New Zealand I've done a lot of reading, spoken to coaches, and closely analyzed all my performances. I've concluded not only that I need to work diligently on and improve my swim times, but also that there's a little room for improvement in my bike and run times, as well as in my transition times from swim to bike and bike to run. It's clear to me now where I need to focus my efforts.

Similarly, when you take on a new position in physical therapy, such as managing a department or facility, you must be aware of gaps in your expertise. Do you understand all of the pertinent financial indicators? Are you good at developing relationships with staff and patients? Are you strong in marketing? How deep is your knowledge of Medicare rules and regulations? The key is to assess yourself honestly early on, to ensure that both you and the department or facility are getting the expertise you need in order to thrive.

Change. If I hope to "swim with the sharks" in the World Championships (no, not literally!) I cannot continue to do things the way I did them. Before New Zealand, I swam 3 days a week with a masters team. I got fitter, but my form changed very little. As a result, breaking 1:30 in a 100-meter swim was a push for me.

Lately, I've devoted my time to changing my actual swim technique. I'm working with a coach a couple of times a month, and we're focusing almost exclusively on drills—almost no "real" swimming. Concentrating on drills that are designed to reduce "drag" through the water, we've seen a dramatic change. By the end of the first month doing the drills, my 100-meter time had dropped to 1:12—a 20% improvement! (And we're not done yet!) It wouldn't have happened had I merely done more of what I'd been doing before. It required a complete change in how I was going about my training.

In your new position or pursuit in physical therapy, you can't simply do more of what you were doing before. That's one of the most common mistakes new managers make. They are good and dedicated clinicians, so they keep the same caseload—or even increase it—in addition to taking on management responsibilities. The result not only is burnout for the PT, but little prospect for long-term improvement in the department or program because the PT is stretched too thin to be an energetic and innovative leader.

Instead, make some specific changes when you move into the new position. Start a new Day-Timer system, perhaps. Block out specific times in your week to devote energy to a new pursuit—such as identifying and working with a mentor, taking a course, or working on an advanced degree. On a simpler scale, change your office layout, buy a new suit or pantsuit, start reading a different magazine or newspaper that may help you do your job better. Add new elements that help spark creativity. Simply doing more of the same old, same old won't cut it.

Get serious. The World Championships were one of the most motivating events of my life. As soon as they were over, I was raring to go in again! Some of my friends thought I was crazy. Enjoy the off-season, they said (before competitions resume in May). Sleep in, they advised. Watch TV! Eat junk food!

For me, those things weren't options. Champions are made during the off-season, not on race day. If I was going to be serious about competing at a world-class level, I knew I needed to get up at 4:45 am every day and hit the pool, the bike, or the road. Some days—especially in Colorado in winter—the pool feels pretty cold at that time in the morning. On those days I often ask myself, "Would a world-champion triathlete skip a workout because the water was a little chilly?" You know the answer to that as well as I do. If that's my vision, it's also an easy answer.

If you're ready to step onto a new playing field as a manager or program developer, you've got a decision to make. Are you willing to get serious? Are you sure you want it? Answer those questions before taking the plunge, because when the need for extra preparation starts and the long hours kick in, it's going to be tempting to give in to mediocrity, to let the little things slide—until all that sliding has left you downhill, looking up. Ask yourself, "Would a world-class manager put off until tomorrow his or her response to that one last e-mail that really should be answered today?" You know the answer to that one, too.

Is this the year that you step up to a new level of performance in pursuing your professional goals? Are you ready to assess, change, and get serious? Put those three legs of your own professional triathlon into place, and you're likely to look back on this year as a championship one. See you at the pool!

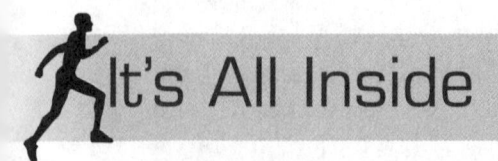

It's All Inside

Try to tap the talents within yourself and others.

My oldest daughter, Ashley, is 10 years old at this writing. One weekend recently, she and I brought our swimsuits to church and headed directly to the pool afterward, as we often do, which eliminates the chance that daddy will spend the entire afternoon in an easy chair with the TV remote.

On this particular day, something happened. Something amazing. Something eye-opening. Something memorable. Something from which we can all learn. Ashley discovered a gift.

To put this analogy in context, you need to know something about Ashley. While I'm clearly prejudiced, she is one of the sweetest little girls you'll ever meet. She has a sensitive heart that consistently picks up on the needs of those around her. She's compassionate, caring, and willing to share anything—her last piece of gum with her 5-year-old brother, her favorite earrings with her younger sister. She's a peacemaker and a compromiser.

But until that weekend, she was not an athlete. That just was not her. She wasn't one to push herself. She always was the first to tire and lag during family hikes, the first to walk her bike up hills during rides. She'd simply watch as her younger sister passed her. No matter how much we'd encourage her, she'd tend to let up, rarely pushing herself. Until the day in question.

Having only recently taken up swimming, Ashley rarely had swum more than 100 meters—four lengths of the pool—at a stretch. On this day, however, she decided she was going to test herself; I never said a word. She told me she thought she might be able to do 400 meters if she took it slow and easy.

As it turned out, she was wrong. She swam 1,000 meters—40 lengths—without stopping a single time. Not once during that time did I say anything remotely related to, "C'mon, just one more." She did it all on her own. Completely. And next time, she says, she wants to do even more.

So, what does that have to do with physical therapists (PTs) and physical therapist assistants (PTAs)? With our facilities? With our careers? Everything!

Our long-term success correlates very closely to the extent to which our hearts are in our work. I'll take an employee with a great attitude and utter devotion to his or her personal growth over someone with natural talent but no drive toward excellence. And I'd guess most of you would, too. We talk about motivating ourselves and our coworkers, but the most effective long-term motivation comes from within—from identifying our gifts and passions, then acting on opportunities to develop and unleash them.

> I'll take an employee with a great attitude and utter devotion to his or her personal growth over someone with natural talent but no drive toward excellence.

For several years I'd been trying, with very limited success, to encourage Ashley to "go for it"—to push herself. Basically, I was trying to make her into me, which is a common error among managers, spouses, and parents. But it was only when she found her heart, her gift, her niche, that she took her efforts to that next level. Why can't we apply the same principle to our facilities and careers? We can! Get started by asking yourself the following questions:

- If you're a supervisor, are you attuned to the special gifts and passions of each of your employees? If not, who's the first one with whom you're going to sit down and discuss those things this week? In his book *The Four Obsessions of the Extraordinary Executive*,[1] Patrick Lencioni advocates a 90-minute performance evaluation of each staffer, because "When you run out of things to talk about, it's then that you talk about what's really important." That's a good lesson for all of us.

- This isn't a one-way street. Team members, wouldn't it be great to work for a motivated supervisor? What are your supervisor's gifts? Could you help relieve her of some responsibilities in areas where she doesn't shine in order to give her time to exercise her special talents? It's likely that everyone will benefit from the results.

- Is there one particular employee whose work is dragging? Who seems disconnected, somehow? Maybe it's not a work issue; maybe he just needs a little extra sleep and a healthier breakfast to start off the day. But then again, perhaps helping him recapture his passion by giving him a chance to exercise his particular gifts would springboard him to renewed vitality.

In *Now, Discover Your Strengths*,[2] Marcus Buckingham cites a Gallup poll that asked those surveyed, "Do you have a chance to do what you do well every day?" Only 20% of the respondents, he notes, "strongly agreed" that they have such an opportunity. Only 20% could honestly say, in other words, that on a daily basis they can use their gift, fulfill their niche, do the one thing they are most urgently motivated to do.

How about you? How would you respond to the Gallup question? What does your answer suggest you need to do today?

References
1. Lencioni PM. *The Four Obsessions of an Extraordinary Executive*. San Francisco: Jossey-Bass; 2000.
2. Buckingham M, Clifton DO. *Now, Discover Your Strengths*. New York, NY: Free Press; 2001.

Subduing 'the Q'

Do you ever feel like quitting? Of course you do! The realization can be freeing.

As I write these words, this is my 13th year as a husband, 11th as a parent, third as a triathlete, and 40th on this Earth. I've experienced many special moments and absorbed some great lessons in all that time. This spring, I was fortunate to learn what just might be the most important lesson of all.

I realized that in most every endeavor—athletic competition, marriage, parent/child relationship, fill in the blank—a specific, identifiable, less-than-welcome moment will come. At some point, the desire to quit—I call it "the Q"—will rear its ugly head.

You read that right. The urge to stop. Let up. Give up. Go home. Give in.

As a husband, quitting time may follow the umpteenth round of a disagreement my wife and I have been having for years. As a parent, it may come in the wake of a teary-eyed, logic-absent discussion with my soon-to-be-teenage daughter. As a triathlete, it's that point in every single race when my head—not to mention my lungs, my legs, and seemingly every other body part—screams, "Enough! I'm done!"

So what, Brad? Why is that such a critical lesson? What difference can recognizing the Q possibly make in your life?

Thanks for asking! It's a critical lesson because I now realize the Q is always coming, always on the way. As a result, I expect it. It's not a surprise, and it no longer causes me anxiety. Once it shows up, I'm ready for it. And the steps I've devised to deal with it make all the difference in the final outcome.

Anytime you push yourself outside your comfort zone, the Q will show up. So stop being surprised when it does.

A Moment-ous Decision

As physical therapists (PTs) and physical therapist assistants (PTAs), we've been through a great deal of change over the past decade or so. Changes in Medicare reimbursement, the (re)emergence of referral for profit (including physician-owned physical therapy services), and the rise and fall (and rise again) of many large health care organizations have tossed some of our best-laid plans out the window. Add to those industry-wide phenomena all the daily changes many of us face with our individual companies, co-workers, and bosses. Throw in personal, family, and societal upheaval, and it sometimes can feel like our backs are against the wall. There may be the temptation to throw in the towel and quit.

One day 2 years ago, that's exactly what I did. Oh, don't worry—Suzanna and I are still together, and the kids still can count on me coming home at night. I didn't go AWOL from my job. Rather, during a Half-Ironman triathlon (1.2-mile swim, 56-mile bike race, 13.1-mile run) 2 years ago in Boulder, Colorado, I walked off the course. I outright quit. I just gave up.

Oh, I had my reasons, and in the literal heat of the moment, they made perfect sense. But, looking back, that decision brings only regret. For those of you who know me, it won't come as any surprise that I'd built this race up in my head as the be-all, end-all of personal athletic achievement. It was the first step in my 3-step "road to Kona" (the Ironman world championships in Hawaii). It was a hot day, and, after leaving a little too much out there on the bike portion of the event, I hit the run needing to average just over 6 minutes per mile for the half-marathon run in order to keep alive my goal of qualifying for Kona. But I ran my first mile in 7 minutes. My next mile dropped to 8 minutes, and I hit the end of the first loop—the halfway point—running somewhere around 9-minute miles, feeling like my legs were wrapped in cement.

So, I quit. I sat right down in front of my entire family and gave up. I still regret it. My wife and kids hardly said a word to me about it then—and still don't talk about it—but I couldn't help but feel, as I looked at them, that I'd simply given in and settled for mediocrity. My resolve began then and there to look inward and figure out why I did what I did, and how I could prevent myself from doing it again.

Delaying Tactics

What I've come to realize is that, in the midst of stress, we must learn to "quiet the Q" if we're to be successful over the long haul. The following are three simple steps to do just that.

Expect it. Anytime you push yourself outside your comfort zone, the Q will show up. So stop being surprised when it does. You don't get startled by the sun coming up each morning; in fact, you plan your day around it. If you view the Q as a difficult road that you've successfully navigated in the past, rather than as a scary curve that may pitch you into a ditch, you're that much more likely to reach your finish line.

"Add two." In a race, when the Q hits, I simply say to myself, "Okay, here it is. Let's just try to hold pace for 2 minutes." Before I know it, those 2 minutes have passed, and my ability to successfully hold off the Q feeds on itself, spurring me on. If your Q is work-related, maybe try holding on for an additional 2 more months while you take steps to make things better. If it's your marriage, perhaps 2 years and commensurate effort. The key is to move your ultimate decision outside the sphere of the Q. Don't make a decision in the heat of the Q.

Analyze. After every race, I look back on the Q and go over with my coach my reactions and responses. With the kids or in our marriage, Suzanna and I discuss the Q moments after things have calmed down—when quitting no longer seems like the answer. Once you've moved past the Q, sit down with your significant other, a mentor, a friend, or a coach to review that crunch moment and learn from the experience—knowing that with the Q, there's always going to be a next time.

To Hold or to Fold?

There may come a time in any aspect of life when making a reasoned decision to pack it in and go in a different direction is appropriate. I'd never advise anyone to stay in a race at clear risk to his or her long-term health, to remain in a job that holds no conceivable promise of better days, to hold fast in an irreparable marriage. But the time to make those kinds of decisive determinations is not in the heat of the Q. That's why it's so vitally important to subdue the Q at such times. To instead look at the ABCs of the situation. Maybe, in some cases, catch some Zs on it.

Then, when you're rested and ready, see if you aren't, in fact, ready to run that next mile after all.

Going the Distance—and Then Some

You can use these two techniques to overcome professional and personal barriers.

I'm passionate about fitness and always get excited when I see others arise from their sedentary lifestyles and begin working out. It's not unusual for people from my professional or personal life to ask my advice about how best to get in shape—or, if they're already physically active, how best to improve their performance. Not long ago, a friend sought me out.

> I had him buy a "super abs" video, a supplement that's guaranteed to cut fat while you sit at your desk, and a starter kit for an Atkins-style diet, right?

He was in his mid-40s and, like so many people, was significantly overweight. (In his case, by about 30 pounds.) He came to me realizing that with each passing year, he was going to find it harder and harder to turn the corner and get fit. "I'm ready to do what I need to do," he said, looking at me expectantly.

So, I had him buy a "super abs" video, a supplement that's guaranteed to cut fat while you sit at your desk, and a starter kit for an Atkins-style diet, right?

Of course not. As any health care professional knows, such steps generally are going to eat into your wallet long before they trim your waistline. You might see minor results at the start, but in the long run such "get-thin-quick" (and easily!) schemes are bound to fail because they tend to change spending habits rather than lifestyles.

So, what did my friend and I really do first?

We created a vision. We went after the "why." Why did he care about the 30 pounds? Much of the population is carrying around excess weight. Why did it matter to him that he was on the heavy side?

His answer was immediate: his children. He's crazy about his kids and is a very involved dad. He's also a health care provider, so he knew the statistics: The possibility of heart disease, diabetes, and a plethora of other scary medical conditions rise exponentially as the waistline expands. He didn't want his weight to cut into the amount of time he has with his family. He envisioned a future spent interacting with his family. My role was helping him get to that vision.

It's been said that if you have a big enough "why," you always can create the "how." Now that he had identified the why, we could move on to the how.

Take the Leap

My friend recalled how he had been a runner back in high school 30 years earlier. He told me that he wanted to try going back to that sport, having heard friends his age talk about running 10Ks, doing marathons, even completing triathlons. So, we set up a training program and got started, right?

Wrong. We went back to the concept of vision. I wanted him to see himself running a 5K race, holding that image up as a goal in his mind's eye. I asked him to pick out an upcoming 5K, send in the registration fee, and mark the date on his calendar. Now he was ready to train. We collaborated on a balanced program designed to ease him into training and prepare him for the big day.

Then, 6 weeks into the training program, I told him it was time to "jump three." What's that? It's an outstanding tool for achieving new levels of performance.

Have you ever heard of an "over-distance" workout? That's where a runner purposely overshoots the race distance during training in order to make the race distance seem comparatively manageable. An individual training for a 10K might run 8 or 10 miles so that running the 10K's 6.2 miles feels comfortably do-able, mentally as well as physically. Jump three follows the same principle, but the "extra mileage" is in the person's head. Let me explain.

"Jump three" continues the vision thread. It involves looking ahead three additional steps in your goals, which has the effect of making the immediate goal feel less intimidating. So, even before the 5K took place, I asked my friend to identify and sign up for three more athletic events of ascending length—a 10K, a 10-mile race, and a half-marathon (13.1 miles). With those races in the back of his mind, the upcoming 5K (3.1 miles) began to seem like little more than a speed bump along the way to his more ambitious goals. His perspective changed, he started challenging himself more during workouts, and his mental focus improved. As I write this column, he's well on his way to what I'm certain will be a strong 5K performance.

Bring It Home

Now, let's relate these concepts to your particular situation. Where can a PT apply the over-distance and jump three principles? Just about anywhere!

Let's say, for example, that you're struggling to keep up with an overloaded schedule. Choose one day during the week on which to do an "over-distance workout"—schedule more patients than you usually would, and accept that that day likely will be busier and longer than are most. When you resume a more-normal schedule the next day, you'll likely find that things seem to be flowing more smoothly and less stressfully than they have been lately. Continue that pattern weekly, and in no time your schedule will be caught up.

Regarding jump three, consider your professional life. Say you're a brand-new PT, fresh out of school, and you're a bit intimidated by the prospect of taking on a full caseload of orthopedic patients. First of all, welcome aboard! But next, "jump three" and think about where you want to be professionally 3 years from now. Do you see yourself running the clinic? Do you envision yourself being board certified in orthopedics? Put those goals on your radar screen and your perspective on that caseload is bound to change for the better.

The potential applications of these techniques are virtually endless, and employing them will benefit your patients while they're benefiting you. In fact, you're probably already using over-distance in your interactions with patients, asking them to perform specific activities at a level that will make standard function seem comparatively easy. Consider introducing jump three concepts as well—focusing on big, long-term goals as well as incremental, shorter-term ones—and you're likely to see less mental resistance, greater compliance, and lower cancellation rates.

Over-distance and jump three techniques really can work for you in both your professional and your personal life. Try them today, with yourself or a patient, and let me know how it goes!

Personality Rules!

Appreciate the Differences!

Many benefits flow from understanding and valuing people's differing temperaments.

A dysfunction has been sweeping the country. It has reached major proportions in the workplace and even in our personal lives, but no physical therapist has ever received a referral for its treatment. It's the "Be Like Me Syndrome," as coined by educational psychologist Linda Berens.[1]

Do you recognize it? You've got this dysfunction if your approach to work and life can be summed up: "Treat patients like I do. Interact with them like I do. Do everything the way I do it, because if I do it that way, it must be the best way for you to do it, too. Right?"

Wrong! We all have different ways of doing and responding to things. Striving to understand—and, better yet, appreciate—these differences can do wonders for our relationships with clients, co-workers, family members, and friends.

Years ago, my wife and I would sit down at the dinner table and talk about what had happened at our workplaces that day. Every once in a while, she would share some office problem with me. After listening to her description, I would immediately (before I learned my lesson) break into my speech about how she could resolve that dilemma if only she would follow my "five easy steps."

Fortunately, I have a very understanding wife, so she let this go for a while. Eventually, however—as I was again describing my five-point strategy—she stopped me mid-sentence and said, "Honey, I love you. But I don't want your solutions—I just want a hug!"

Have you been there? Most likely, the answer is yes! We spend our time following the Golden Rule, treating others the way *we* want to be treated. Instead, we need to pursue what the business press calls the "platinum rule," and treat others the way *they* want to be treated. In order to do so, however, we need to have a better understanding of the differences between people as well as a clearer understanding of our own preferences.

Four Types

The notion that people are born with fundamentally different temperaments or predispositions to act in certain ways dates all the way back to the ancient Greeks, but only in the last half-century have behavioral scientists intensively studied these differences. (There's a good summary of the development of "temperament theory" in David Keirsey's *Please Understand Me II*,[2] an updated and greatly expanded edition of his 1978 bestseller *Please Understand Me*.[3])

In 1962, Isabel Myers and her mother, Kathryn Briggs, published the Myers-Briggs Type Indicator (available on the Internet at www.myers-briggs-type-indicator.com), a widely used questionnaire that is designed to identify the user's personality type. As someone who speaks nationwide on such topics as customer focus and teamwork, I've employed my background as a qualified

CHARACTERISTICS OF THE FOUR TEMPERAMENTS

	Idealist	Rational	Guardian	Artisan
Need	Unique Identity	Competence	Belonging	Freedom
Interacts Through	Recognition	Knowledge	Service	Impact
Communication Style	Dramatic	Scholarly	Factual	Colorful
Communicates With	Metaphors, Universals	Conditionals, Precise Definitions	Comparatives, Measurements	Anecdotes, Questions
At Work, Promotes	Growth	Efficiency	Structure	Opportunity
Professional Focus	Ideas & Causes	Ideals & Models	People—Care-taking Services	People—Impacting
Leads By	Giving Praise	Developing Strategies	Administering	Taking Action
Best Environment	Expressive/Personal	Innovative/Intellectual	Organized/Secure	Stimulating/Variety
Stressors	Betrayal	Incompetence	Insubordination	Boredom
Motto	"To Thine Own Self Be True"	"Be Excellent In All Things"	"Early to Bed, Early to Rise"	"Carpe Diem"

(Adapted from Berens LV. *Understanding Yourself and Others: An Introduction to Temperament.* Huntington Beach, Calif: Temperament Research Institute; 1998:24-25. Used with permission.)

Myers-Briggs Type Indicator facilitator to examine temperament differences within groups of varying sizes.

A simple analogy that captures the essence of temperament comes from the aforementioned Linda Berens. In *Understanding Yourself and Others—An Introduction to Temperament*,[4] she explains that our personalities are very much like varieties of trees. Just as a pine cone will not grow into an oak tree and an acorn will not produce a pine tree, a person with one type of temperament won't grow into an adult with a different type of personality. (And just as there are many varieties within the same type of tree, Berens notes—because of differences in soil, water, and available sunlight—so, too, are there variations, related to upbringing and social factors, among people who share the same general temperament.)

In their books, Keirsey (whose Keirsey Temperament Sorter incorporates ideas from Myers-Briggs) and Berens outline the properties of four basic temperaments or personality types—Artisan, Guardian, Rational, and Idealist. (These designations go back to Plato; again, Keirsey[2] is a good background source.) Everyone has aspects of all four temperaments, but temperament theory holds that each person fits squarely within the broad outlines of one or the other. I'll only scratch the surface here in describing these types, but hopefully this introduction will start you and the team of people with whom you work on a journey of discovery.

The ***Artisan*** seeks options and variation in his or her work and play, and feels compelled to produce results and make an impact. Artisans tend to trust their impulses, thinking they can solve any problem they run into. They are excellent negotiators and gifted tacticians. They need the space to pursue their own approaches, but they tend to get results when they're granted that freedom.

The ***Guardian*** embodies predictability. Guardians strongly value accountability and responsibility. They will generously give of their time and resources in order to help keep things running smoothly. Guardians keep a close eye on tradition, as they value security and stability. They are gifted at ensuring that things are "done right."

The ***Rational*** person deftly employs logic and reasoning skills and can be a skillful inventor. Precision is very important to him or her, as is having a solid rationale for every decision. The most successful participants on TV's *Who Wants To Be a Millionaire?* undoubtedly have a rational temperament (and perhaps a bit of a lucky streak).

The ***Idealist*** places his or her greatest emphasis on authenticity (being oneself) and on finding the true meaning in things. Idealists are empathetic and benevolent, and they tend to trust their intuition. They are drawn toward pursuits that expand other people's personal growth. Making the world a better place is at the top of the Idealist's priority list.

A Combustible Mix

Can you see any potential problems when these various temperaments meet in the workplace? Let's say, for example, that someone with a Guardian temperament runs a physical therapy clinic or department that includes people who have the other three temperaments. Mindless of her staff's preferences, the Guardian manager may impose step-by-step procedures for doing things "just right."

What's wrong with that? We need structure in our facilities, don't we—especially with the tight regulations that govern physical therapy? But what happens when the Guardian approach is taken to the extreme? How will team members with other preferences respond to that scenario?

Let's start with the Idealist. Remember, empathy and the primacy of interpersonal relationships are what Idealists are all about. It's unlikely, however, that the extreme Guardian leader will devote nearly as much time to monitoring the team's personal interactions with the patient/client as he or she will expend on ensuring that everything is procedurally going according to plan. Similarly, it's unlikely that the Guardian leader will praise the Idealist simply for admirably performing tasks that the Guardian views as essential and basic. While Guardians don't purposely ignore others' feelings, such sensitivity often takes a back seat to adhering to rules and regulations. If this pattern sets in, the Idealist—who may be an extremely valuable employee—may become disillusioned to the point of seeking another employer.

The Rational person, meanwhile, has a natural talent for inventing things and for long-range planning and strategizing. How well will those skills be nurtured when the Guardian who is running the department or clinic insists on doing everything strictly by the book? Rational people must be allowed to think for themselves, and they seek support for goals and plans that may not have an immediate payoff. The Rational person will quickly come to resent an office structure that inhibits his or her ability to strategize and implement new and better ways of doing things.

Then there's the Artisan. Look back at that person's core need for plenty of options in his or her approach to work and play. Physical therapy already is loaded down with restrictions imposed by insurance company rules, governmental programs, and physicians. How long do you think a person with an Artisan temperament will stick around the clinic if his or her Guardian manager only adds to those restrictions and offers the Artisan no freedom to practice in ways he or she thinks best?

(I want to add here that I'm using the example of an "extreme" Guardian in this column for illustrative purposes only. I don't want to paint a negative picture of people who have this temperament. Because Guardians tend to excel at keeping everything on track, they're extremely important to physical therapy. They help ensure that procedures are followed by the book and that meticulous records are kept—key attributes in a highly regulated profession.)

It Takes All Kinds

Is the Guardian manager's best solution, then, to hire only those who are just like her? If the word "yes" flashed across your mind for even an instant, you're not only on the wrong path—you're on the wrong continent! Absolutely, positively, NO! Lose the variety of temperaments and you lose those individuals' strengths as well. And the truth is, there's no "right" temperament for managers to have; there are successful leaders of each type. Successful leaders have one thing in common, though: They value and get the most out of people with *all* types of temperaments.

As you review the chart on page 104 and think about where you fit in, consider how the Guardian manager could most effectively assimilate the strengths of staff members with temperaments different from her own—and avoid wasting energy, creating ill will, and diminishing potential returns by attempting to force square pegs into round holes.

The Artisan. Artisans often are brimming with innovative ideas, they're willing to take risks, and they can be invaluable in dealing with unexpected situations. The Guardian manager would do well to solicit and heed the Artisan's suggestions—particularly when the by-the-book approach isn't working. The wise Guardian knows that unforeseen circumstances sometimes require unanticipated approaches; the Artisan can be masterful at crafting them.

The Idealist. Because Idealists are empathetic and place great emphasis on interpersonal relationships, the Guardian PT leader might consider tapping the staff Idealist to take a lead role in addressing patient/client concerns or in coordinating a community service/outreach program.

The Rational person. As noted previously, the Rational individual can be great at coming up with new and better ways of doing things. The smart Guardian leader will not only hear out but also seek out the Rational staff member's ideas for making procedures more efficient and effective, because people with the Rational temperament tend to be well-read in the latest literature and know what's working within the profession.

One of the critical things to remember is that we all can—and do—function outside of our natural temperaments, or preferences, at times. Life requires that. You'll notice, however, that whenever you function within your preferences things seems to require less energy and come a little easier.

The key is to help those around you to spend as much time functioning inside their preferences as possible. This is as true for family members as it is for co-workers and clients. If you can tune into people's temperaments, the results can be fantastic: improved bottom-line results, enhanced customer service, heightened energy in your facility, less turnover, and happier families of employees who work with and for you. Wouldn't you say all that is worth considering?

References
1. Berens LV, Ernst L, Robb J, Smith M. *Temperament and Type Dynamics: The Facilitator's Guide*. Huntington Beach, Calif: Telos Publications; 1998.
2. Keirsey D. *Please Understand Me II*. Del Mar, Calif: Prometheus Nemesis Book Company; 1998.
3. Keirsey D, Bates M. *Please Understand Me*. Del Mar, Calif: Prometheus Nemesis Book Company; 1978.
4. Berens, LV. *Understanding Yourself and Others: An Introduction to Temperament*. Huntington Beach, Calif: Temperament Research Institute; 1998.

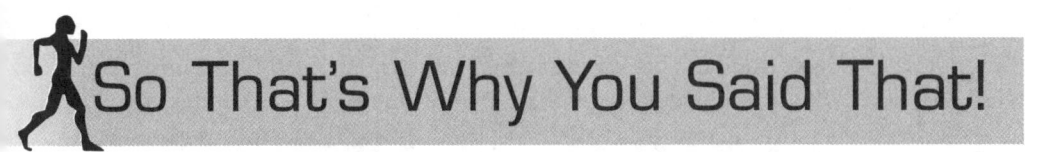

So That's Why You Said That!

Understanding interaction styles can make you a more effective professional.

"He's a *jerk*!"

"She never says *anything* in meetings."

"She has *no* idea that what she said hurt my feelings."

"Why would he *say* that?"

It's all too common: Someone makes a comment that never was intended to cause a rift in a relationship, only to find out months later that it has. This doesn't happen only in relationships with peers or supervisors. It also may be happening in your dealings with your clients, your patients, and the physicians with whom you work.

Does it have to be that way? No. Now, admittedly, some people just don't care about the vibes they give off. They may even go out of their way to flaunt their disgruntled disposition. Most people, however, want to get along with their co-workers, their clients, and their friends. We all have very different interaction styles, though, and the ways in which we relate to other people affect how we get along with them.

A little understanding of the ways in which we interrelate can make a big difference in governing our actions, with both short-term and professional implications. Let's take a look at some of the distinct differences in interaction styles so that you can identify and appreciate them—and see the similarities among them, too.

What's Your Style?

In her book *The 16 Personality Types: Descriptions for Self-Discovery*,[1] educational psychologist Linda Berens describes two major ways in which human interactions begin and two major ways in which they are conducted. The first two are "responding" and "initiating," and the latter two are "directing" and "informing."

Let's start with the ways in which interactions begin. Think about the last time you went to a meeting where you knew very few people—perhaps you recently attended APTA's Annual Conference for the first time, for example. Did you initiate interaction by going up to people, introducing yourself, and starting conversations? Or did you sit back, browse through the information packet, and mostly respond to people who started conversations with you?

	Directing	Informing
Responding	Chart the Course	Behind the Scenes
Initiating	In Charge	Get Things Going

(Source: Cooper B, Berens L. *Groundbreaking Sales Skills: Portable Sales Techniques to Ensure Success.* Huntington Beach, Calif: Telos Publications; 2004. Used with permission.)

Your answer says a great deal about your interaction style. If you initiated conversations, you probably have an external focus and tend to reach out to interact with those around you. If you waited for others to initiate conversations with you, on the other hand, you likely have more of an internal focus, and may well be a more reflective type of person. Neither of these interaction styles is good or bad. They just "are."

Let's move on to the ways in which interactions are conducted. What would you say, for example, if you ran out of ultrasound gel in your clinic (assuming you weren't filling the orders yourself, of course). Would you inform the appropriate staff person: "Joe, we're out of ultrasound gel"? or would you direct: "Joe, you need to order some more gel"?

Both statements can be modified and softened. The first, for example, might be restated: "Joe, we're out of ultrasound gel and it's very important that we have more in by next week." The second could be made into a question and expressed in a gentler way: "Joe, would you please order some more ultrasound gel?" Even

Section 5 — Personality Rules!

with those adjustments, however, in the first case you're informing Joe and in the latter instance you're directing him to do something.

Listen to yourself through the course of the day and consider your own preference. While you may sometimes inform and at other times direct, it's very likely that you favor one interaction style over the other.

Now let's pull together all of the interaction styles I've been describing—initiating, responding, directing, and informing—and examine the various ways in which they fit together and where you fit in the chart on page 109.

As you look at the chart, select your preference on each axis and see where the two preferences meet. For example, if you tend to respond and direct, you fall into the overall interaction style titled "Chart the Course." If you lean, instead, toward informing and initiating, then your overall interaction style is to "Get Things Going."

Before I further describe these designations (as outlined in Berens' *The Guide for Facilitating the Self-Discovery Process*[2]), let me stress, again, that no one designation is better than the others. Sometimes those in management positions, for example, feel they need to be more "In Charge." But many wonderful managers operate quite effectively in the "Behind the Scenes" style. The key is to understand what your preferences are, and to learn to use your strengths and understand how others' preferences may be different from your own.

Choosing It

The following are key characteristics of the four interaction designations Berens describes in *The Guide for Facilitating the Self-Discovery Process:*

Chart the Course. Individuals with this interaction style foresee, analyze, conceptualize, or plan. They explain, but direct only when the necessary action is not taken. They focus on having a plan of action and then moving people along according to that plan.

Behind the Scenes. Individuals with this interaction style focus on designing, composing, and supporting. "Behind the Scenes" people have a talent for enlisting buy-in by concentrating on the quality or soundness of the idea. They focus on integrating everyone's input to get the best possible result.

Get Things Going. People with this style concentrate on helping others explore, discover, and get things accomplished. They act as catalysts by sharing their insights, making preparations, or initiating actions. Their focus is on involving others in the process as much as they possibly can.

In Charge. Those with this style initiate and direct others to accomplish goals. They quickly see what needs to happen and then make it so by mobilizing, supervising, mentoring, and expediting the action of others. Their overriding focus is on getting things done.

In addition to thinking about which of these designations best describes you, you might try soliciting the feedback of others and seeking guidance from a qualified Myers-Briggs facilitator. You can gain further insight into your personal preferences by reading "Appreciate the Differences," (see page 103), which looks at the different types of temperaments people have.

Applying It

Once you have a good handle on which designation fits you best, you can apply this awareness to the way you go about your daily tasks. Here are some examples:

Selecting (and accepting) assignments. Are the projects you take on in sync with the interaction designation that best describes you? For example, if you're a "Behind the Scenes" type of person but as a manager you've tried to mimic a former supervisor's "In Charge" style, you might find yourself uncomfortable with that choice. It's not you—it's a bad fit, style-wise! Instead, try approaching projects in a manner that's more in keeping with your true style. You're likely to be happier and get better results.

Giving assignments. Obviously what's true for you is also true for the people who report to you or work around you. Have you considered their style before giving them assignments? Doing so is likely to positively affect their productivity and reduce procrastination.

Marketing. Have you considered interaction styles in terms of marketing? It's worth a thought! Look for clues when you meet with potential clients. Even if you can't quite discern their interaction style or temperament, the fact that you're looking for it will make you a better listener. If you do pick up on clues, try to mimic the client's style somewhat. For example, if a person appears to be more of an informing/responding ("Behind the Scenes") type, provide a lot of information and slowly introduce some choices he or she might want to consider. And don't rush into things with a directing/initiating ("In Charge") type of person—if you do, you're likely to turn off that individual very quickly. People like working with those they perceive as being like themselves. Making some effort along those lines can help you forge better relationships with others.

Building teams. Discussing interaction styles with the other members of your office team can be very valuable in helping everyone understand and appreciate each other's preferences. The discussion that might ensue from introducing these concepts into the group could go a long way toward building a better and more cohesive team!

It's certainly true that interaction styles don't always fit into nice, neat boxes. We all have components of various styles, and we may interact differently depending on the circumstances and situation. Everyone has prevailing tendencies, though. The better your understanding of yourself and others in relation to these basics, the better your chances at effective interaction with those around you!

References
1. Berens LV, Nardi D. *The 16 Personality Types: Descriptions for Self-Discovery.* Huntington Beach, Calif: Telos Publications; 1999.
2. Berens LV, Ernst L, Smith M. *The Guide for Facilitating the Self-Discovery Process.* Huntington Beach, Calif: Temperament Research Institute; 2000.

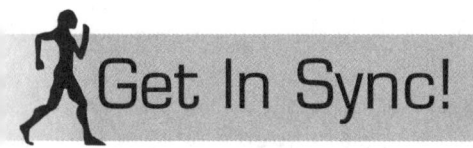

Get In Sync!

Physical therapists who match their "sales approach" to the temperaments of the people to whom they're "selling" their services and products are more likely to be successful in achieving desired results.

Physical therapists (PTs) are constantly "selling" on some level. They primarily sell their services—their knowledge and skills, both in and of themselves and in comparison with those of their competitors. Sometimes they're selling to physicians, at other times to patients/clients, sometimes even to coworkers. Many PTs in private practice also sell products that are beneficial to their patients/clients, such as exercise equipment, through their clinics.

One of the goals of any PT—and the entrepreneurial PT in particular—is to build trust, curiosity, and interest in your services so that your business grows. Within that simple goal, however, are a number of variables, one of which is the need to connect with the client (and here I'm using "client" in a general sense, not just as in the term "patient/client"). If that connection isn't made, success at the next level (the "sale") is considerably less likely.

It isn't news that individuals tend to connect with people they see as being similar to themselves—having the same interests and congruent backgrounds. One of the basic pointers in any sales training course is the importance of finding conversational topics through which to establish common ground with the client. But what if you could go deeper? What if you could pick up on traits that would point you toward their temperament and core needs.

Before I go any further, please realize that the advice I'm about to give is only a starting point. Getting a clear reading on your own temperament and how you naturally interact with others can take time. Ideally, you should meet with a qualified facilitator and perhaps use the Myers-Briggs Type Indicator (more information at www.myers-briggs-type-indicator.com). The advice that follows offers some hints about people's temperaments and how to most effectively interact with each temperament type, but you shouldn't extrapolate all this too far without looking into it further. Still, studying these tips may well enhance your interactions with both potential and current clients.

First, take a look at the descriptions in the box on this page. These are the four basic temperaments or personality types, as I describe them in "Appreciate the Differences!" (see page 103). As I explained in that piece, the notion that people are born with fundamentally different temperaments or predispositions to act in certain ways dates all the way back to the ancient Greeks, but only in the last half-century have behavioral scientists intensively studied these differences. The four basic personality types described in the box are explored in greater detail in the work of David Keirsey[1,2] (whose Keirsey Temperament Sorter incorporates ideas from Myers-Briggs) and Linda Berens.[3] Those books offer greater insight into where the people to whom you're selling "fit," temperamentally.

Now, let's look at some keys to connecting with people who have each of these four personality types—a process I call "sync selling."

The Artisan

To begin with, it's important to realize that an Artisan may have a somewhat cynical point of view toward your services or products, with the thought that you're only in it for your purposes, not his or hers. With that in mind, it is extremely important that you make a connection early on with the Artisan, before distrust has a chance to build.

For the Artisan, making a connection begins with the projection of confidence. The Artisan is adept at reading body language; signs of discomfort on your part will be obvious to him or her. If you don't seem sure of yourself and "together" from the outset, your chance of success with the Artisan is minimal.

Ease of process is another way to connect rapidly with the Artisan. Artisans are eager to try something new. Artisan physicians and patients will be very interested, for example, in hearing about "cutting-edge" services at your clinic. They're unlikely, however, to be interested in spending much time dwelling on the background and details. Impress the Artisan from the outset with enthusiastic "bullet points," and your chances of success will increase significantly. By the same token, however, the Artisan's tendency toward quick decisions may turn against you if

"Sales" Strategies

The "general" tips below apply to anyone of that temperament to whom you're selling. Many of the "ideas" apply more specifically to physicians.

The Artisan	The Guardian	The Idealist	The Rational Person
General:	General:	General:	General:
• Emphasize flash and impact.	• Emphasize stability, security.	• Ensure that the person can relate to you.	• Firmly establish your credentials from the outset.
• Provide a multitude of negotiating options.	• Just the facts—no fluff.	• Avoid overstating.	• Provide research on why your services and products are the best option for him or her.
Some ideas:	Some ideas:	Some ideas:	
• Host quick, spur-of-the-moment meetings.	• Schedule a meeting several weeks in advance.	• Gradually move from "helping," to "introducing," to "showing," to "selling."	Some ideas:
• Get out of the office (golf, lunch, etc).	• Bring literature that attests to the stability of your clinic and the dependability of your services and products.	• Engage in relationship-building activities such as going out to lunch—and stay away from sales talk at such times.	• Offer an educational seminar.
• Provide demonstrations but keep them brief (promise 5 minutes—use 3 and you'll have a fan).	• Keep it simple; taking the Guardian out to a fancy lunch, for instance, may be seen as wasteful and even irresponsible.	• Bring into the sales process people with whom the person has a personal relationship, through personal introductions or letters of recommendation.	• Involve the person in a study or focus group, asking his or her suggestions on how the service or product could be enhanced.
			• Leave a pertinent article for the physician to read; give patients/clients a list of Web sites at which their questions might be further addressed.

For more information, see *The Quick Guide to the Four Temperaments and Sales* by Brad Cooper.[4]

you stumble early. The Artisan is ready to take care of business and then move on to the next item. A request for patience or a lengthy dissertation from you is likely to seal your fate.

Impact is key! If you can quickly communicate to the Artisan the short-term impact of your services or products, you'll more likely gain his or her attention. Artisans are of the moment. They generally aren't as intensely interested in what the payoff will be well down the road. Thus, the Artisan physician wants to know how physical therapy can begin helping his or her patient *today*. Similarly, the Artisan patient will be most strongly motivated to follow a home program or purchase needed exercise equipment (if it is not reimbursable by insurance) if you strongly emphasize the immediate benefits he or she is likely to see, and the freedom the product will help him or her achieve.

Also, be prepared to negotiate or debate with the Artisan, or his or her interest in the process may be lost. Artisans generally enjoy the banter of a good give-and-take discussion.

Because Artisans "need space," as per the description in the chart, it's important that you seek out opportunities to create a loosely structured atmosphere and don't move quickly into discussions about details. Give the Artisan patient/client a flexible home program and offer him or her a hand in designing it, rather than presenting it as a long-term commitment that requires him or her to do X, Y, and Z. In selling an Artisan physician on your services, don't try to pin him or her down during a standard office visit. When possible, a brief introductory meeting followed up by some sort of social activity out of the office is likely to be your best bet.

Finally, avoid too much abstraction or wordiness in discussions with the Artisan. The Artisan's mind is quick to wander, and your "sale" could be lost if you are too indirect.

The Guardian

Your best sales route with the Guardian is very different from that taken with the Artisan. Rather than seeking flash and impact, the Guardian is on the lookout for people who are dependable and timely.

Tradition and consistency hold a great deal of value for the Guardian, so an emphasis on "the latest and greatest" is *not* likely to be very effective in this case. Instead, talk about how your services enhance what the Guardian currently has in place. Here's something you might say to a Guardian patient/client: "The last three visits we've been doing joint mobilizations and soft tissue work. I have a technique I'm going to use with you today that will build on what we've been doing and continue your progress." With a Guardian physician, frequent, consistent communication is the key. Suggest that the two of you meet regularly to discuss patients and their progress. The Guardian physician will likely be responsive.

The Guardian looks to common sense and history as his or her guides. What worked in the past? Does the service or product have a record of effectiveness? Emphasize these points—perhaps with pertinent articles or other literature. In addition, because membership in established, respected organizations is important to the Guardian, recommendations of your services from others in his or her "group"—such as other physicians, for instance—can be helpful in guiding his or her decisions.

Guardians are on the other end of the spectrum from the Artisan in their interest in details; discussions of protocols and lists of benefits will be well received. And, because the Guardian has a core need for stability, if that list of benefits includes warranties, customer support, and back-up plans (when you're discussing exercise products, for instance), these will be viewed as valuable selling points.

When it comes to meetings, Guardians prefer specific scheduling, in advance, and you'd better not be late or cancel without considerable advance notice. To the Guardian, tardiness and late cancellations demonstrate a serious lack of respect. If you engage in such behaviors your ability to connect with this person will be severely damaged.

The Idealist

You had best project sincerity if you want to market effectively to the Idealist. The "classic" slick salesperson will be least effective with this individual, who will immediately pick up on (and summarily reject) any form of canned presentation or perceived lack of authenticity.

The Idealist is most concerned about people and helping them reach their potential. Stress this aspect of physical therapy and the products you sell—but tell it from your heart. Share stories of people who personally have seen results—and if your examples are people the Idealist knows, so much the better. Also, empathize, when you can, with what your patients/clients are going through. Talk about back pain that you've had, and how physical therapy helped.

Details such as calling people by name and treating them with warmth and courtesy are certain to be noticed by the Idealist. He or she will take special note of how you interact with everyone—from your own staff to his or her receptionist. If you let up in this area your meeting may be as good as done.

It is very important to establish a personal link with the Idealist. Emphasize some connection that differentiates you from the crowd of competitors and your chances for success will escalate considerably. If it comes out that the potential client is an avid tennis player, for example, and you play tennis, too, engage the Idealist in a conversation about the joys and frustrations of the game. The Idealist may come to think of you as a fellow tennis player who happens to have services to sell, rather than as a seller first.

The Idealist generally will be congenial and will not cut you off. Knowing that, bring extra sensitivity to the table and cut yourself off earlier than you normally might, intentionally allowing him or her time for questions. Your success with a person of this temperament will be based, before all else, on your relationship with and consideration for him or her.

The Rational Person

"How well does it really work?" and "Why does it work so well?" are the types of questions you'll need to address when working with someone of the Rational temperament.

Knowledge and research are foremost for this person. Produce the evidence. Point to germane research about specific interventions or articles about the benefits of physical therapy that recently were published in professional journals, respected newspapers, and magazines. Send over a copy of an article tied to a discussion the two of you have had recently. You might even consider sending the person an abstract directly from a seminar you attended—sharing the "latest information" about a service or product you've been discussing with that person.

Strategy is also a key area to the Rational person. Demonstrate how what you're "selling" serves his or her overall long-term strategy and you'll likely get his or her ear. When you do so, however, be sure that it's *his* or *her* strategy you're addressing, not the strategy *you* think is best. While the Rational person is open to your suggestions, he or she derives pleasure from designing the strategy. In designing an exercise program for a patient/client, after setting the basic rules that the person cannot break, encourage the person to develop his or her own variations on the assigned exercises.

Ask the Rational physician what he or she thinks about a recent study that may hold implications for the patient's care. Invite the Rational physician to participate in an orthopedic study group with your staff.

One final thought: As you might suspect, "warm and fuzzy" approaches are not effective with Rational people. They're interested in the "whys" and "hows." Answer those questions and you'll be well on your way to making the sale.

References
1. Keirsey D. *Please Understand Me II*. Del Mar, Calif: Prometheus Nemesis Book Company; 1998.
2. Keirsey D, Bates M. *Please Understand Me*. Del Mar, Calif: Prometheus Nemesis Book Company; 1978.
3. Berens, LV. *Understanding Yourself and Others: An Introduction to Temperament*. Huntington Beach, Calif: Temperament Research Institute; 1998.
4. Cooper, B. *The Quick Guide to Four Temperaments and Sales*. Hunting Beach, Calif: Telos Publications; 2003.

Greet the Clock

It's About Time

Everyone agrees that there isn't enough of it in a day, but few people do what it takes to manage it effectively. Here are some tips that will help.

Time has become our most valuable commodity. We count on handheld palm computers to guide us through our busy schedules. We favor e-mail over slower fax machines. Pagers and cell phones keep us in touch 24 hours a day. We're all looking for ways to squeeze out extra minutes. The key to having the time to do the things that are the most important to us lies, however, not so much in the use of high-tech devices as in effective overall time management.

You can manage your time more effectively by implementing the strategies I'm about to outline. They include appreciating Stephen Covey's concept of four quadrants of activity, which I first touched on in the pages of *PT Magazine* in 1997[1]; looking closely at your "Nows" and "WOWs"—a concept I discuss more extensively in "Awakening the WOW" (see page 55); and heeding some specific tips on efficient use of the telephone and e-mail.

No less a multitasker than Benjamin Franklin once said, "If time be of all things the most precious, wasting time must be the greatest prodigality." That's as true today as it was in his day, but you needn't be among the worst offenders. So, let's look at some great ways to conserve this extremely precious resource.

Four Quadrants

In Covey's modern-day classic of leadership literature, *The 7 Habits of Highly Effective People*,[2] he divides all the activities of life into four different quadrants.

Quadrant I consists of activities that are urgent and important. Most of these things once resided in Quadrant II, the home of activities that are important but not (yet) urgent. What happens is, Quadrant II activities too often get neglected because of procrastination or too much time spent putting out Quadrant I fires, until they themselves become Quadrant I activities. While you can't expect ever to eliminate Quadrant I—there are always going to be emergencies and unexpected events in your life that demand immediate attention—the more time you spend taking care of business in Quadrant II, the less time and energy you'll have to spend in Quadrant I, away from the things you really want to be doing.

	Urgent	Not Urgent
Important	Quadrant I	Quadrant II
Not Important	Quadrant III	Quadrant IV

Quadrant II is the place to be, but it's tough to get there! Keeping activities in Quadrant II requires that you do things *before* they actually need to be done. This involves planning and self-motivation. It doesn't take much self-motivation to get something done the day it's due—your job's on the line by then! The trick is to motivate yourself to get things done consistently a week before the deadline. This plan not only eliminates the need to rush through activities, but it gives you the time to do them right and complete them on your terms. It puts you in charge. Procrastinating, on the other hand, puts the deadline in charge, instead of you.

There are two other quadrants you can and should shrink or eliminate, leaving you with more time in Quadrant II and increasing your effectiveness over the long haul. They are Quadrant III, in which activities are urgent but not important, and Quadrant IV, a recovery quadrant in which activities are neither urgent nor important.

Quadrant III is where many people end up spending huge portions of their lives, even though they don't mean to. People immersed in Quadrant III are simply responding to a sense of urgency without ever taking a step back to see if the activity is really worth the time it takes to respond.

Consider this example of a Quadrant III activity. You're in the midst of treating a patient or working on an important project, and you get an overhead page that you have a call on line 1. You interrupt your train of thought to take the call, only to find out that the caller is the local linoleum salesman. Nothing against linoleum salesmen, but compared with the Quadrant II activity in which you were engaged, that call simply doesn't stack up! It was "urgent" because you were paged, but it wasn't really important.

Fortunately, however, Quadrant III can be all but eliminated with a little planning. In the case of phone calls, for example, instruct staff not to page you when you're with a patient or involved in another important activity unless the call really should take precedence. And define to staff which types of calls, from whom, *do* take precedence.

Have you ever heard the saying, "Men don't care what's on TV—they just care what *else* is on TV"? Well, that attitude is classic Quadrant IV. There's nothing wrong with spending some time in front of the TV. But the question is, are you watching a particular show because you really enjoy it? That would make it a Quadrant II activity, because it's genuinely important for you to enjoy your "down" time. On the other hand, however, are you just endlessly clicking the remote from one show to the next because you're too exhausted from all the time you've been spending in Quadrants I and III to do anything else? It's easy to see how better planning in and devotion to Quadrant II can dramatically reduce the amount of time you need to spend in Quadrants I and III, eliminating the need for you to recover from the stress by mentally "vegging out" in Quadrant IV.

"Nows" and "WOWs"

But how do you get there? How do you begin spending more time in Quadrant II and less time in Quadrants I, III, and IV? I employ a "Nows and WOWs" system. Here, in a nutshell, is how this system works.

> Throw out the idea of compiling a "to-do" list, because its very name implies that you must do everything on it.

First of all, throw out the idea of compiling a "to-do" list, because its very name implies that you must do everything on it. That's not true! Instead, draw up a "list of possibilities." That name changes the mindset and encourages you to focus on getting the most out of your time.

Now that you've got your list of possibilities, start looking at your Quadrant II activities—things you've deemed important but not urgent—and ask the following questions:

- What on this list is a "WOW"—something that gets your juices flowing and thus requires little self motivation to initiate?
- What on this list is a "Now"—something you might not necessarily enjoy doing, but that needs to be completed in the near future?

- After identifying all the activities that fit into those two categories, you're likely to be left with things that are neither WOWs nor Nows. You've got three options as to how to address these activities:

- You can try to turn them into WOWs by spicing them up and making them cool and desirable. For example, it may be necessary to hold a staff meeting, but you might be dreading it because such meetings tend to be boring. With a little creativity on your part, however—say, inviting a thought-provoking guest speaker or introducing a role-playing game that sparks everyone's creativity—that normally dull gathering can become a big-time WOW!

- Say there are things on your list that need to be done eventually but keep getting put off to the indefinite future. Move up their timetable by a day, a week, or a month. This makes them Nows and puts them higher on your radar screen.

- Determine which of your non-WOW, non-Now activities are simply unimportant, and eliminate them from your list. It turns out they weren't Quadrant II material after all.

By going through this process on a regular basis, you'll put yourself ahead of the game by reducing the number of activities getting shoved into Quadrant I and eliminating unnecessary yet time-consuming Quadrant III and Quadrant IV activities.

The final step is to commit yourself to completing all your Nows before touching your WOWs. Since you look forward to WOW activities, you're sorely tempted to pursue them first. But if you do that, tackling the WOWs when you're fresh and full of energy, the Nows may become leftovers—constantly getting pushed back, edging closer and closer each day to Quadrant I. If, on the other hand, you complete the Now activities earlier in the day, when you're operating on all cylinders, and you use your WOWs as enticements for later in the day, you'll end up being far more effective and productive in the long run.

On the Phone and Online

Think of how much time you spend on the phone and writing and responding to e-mail. Heed the following suggestions, and you'll open up that much more time:

The phone. Always have work-related materials handy to look at while you're on hold. You spend a lot of time over the months waiting for someone to come to the phone or for their voice mail recording to play. If you're doing something productive during all these 30-second interludes, you'll end up saving yourself precious time that might otherwise have been wasted listening to Muzak or yet another "I'm not here" message.

Here are some additional phone tips:

- Before picking up the phone to make or take a call, ask yourself the relative importance of the call, whether it's truly urgent, and if the time you'll spend on the phone will hinder, have little effect on, or enhance your ability to do what you need to do that day.

  If it's urgent and important or will enhance your effectiveness, by all means, make or take the call. If it's not urgent or vitally important, but you can spare the time on the phone without significantly affecting your productivity, you may wish to make or take the call. Assess each case individually. But if the call isn't that important and it would take you further away from achieving your goals, consider simply continuing the Quadrant II activities in which you're engaged and making or returning the call at a time that's better for you.

- Keep a phone log to track your calls. Not only will it remind you of who you need to call back, but you can use it to look at patterns and see if there's anything you can do to reduce your volume of calls.

- Start off the call right! Instead of saying, "Hi, Sue. How are you?"—which is great if you've some got time to chat, but makes little sense if both of you are rushed—begin, "Sue, this is Jan. I know you're busy, but I've got one quick question."

- Finally, plan to return calls at a specific time of day, rather than interrupting your activities and your train of thought constantly throughout the day. Consider using the late afternoon as your phone time. At that point, you're starting to wind down from a busy day, and most phone calls take less energy than your patient visits and special projects.

E-mail. Never leave messages to pile up in your "In box" for more than 48 hours. Read them as promptly as you can and respond as appropriate. It will save you time in the long run if you don't have to sort through lengthy queues of accumulated e-mail messages every several days.

Here's some additional advice for better time management with e-mail:

- When you send messages, include a descriptive subject line. That way, your recipient—who may receive 100 or more e-mail messages a day—will know with just a quick glance why you're writing and may be likelier to respond promptly. The faster people respond to you, the more quickly and efficiently you can get your own work done.

- As with phone calls, consider setting aside a specific time of the day to view and respond to e-mail. Answering messages as they come can distract you from what you're working on and decrease your efficiency.

Section 6 — Greet the Clock **123**

- Keep your messages short and sweet. Keep the "scroll-down rule" in mind. If your message is long enough that the recipient must scroll down to read it all, you may have spent too much time going into too much detail, and the recipient may end up storing it to read later rather than responding quickly.

- Set up your autosignature ahead of time. It takes 5 minutes and saves you the time-consuming chore of having to re-type your name, title, and contact information with each new message you send.

- Watch what you write and how you write it. Remember, you are the message! In today's world, the only thing many people may know about you is how you come across on your e-mail. Poor grammar and word choices reflect negatively on you, and you may not always get an opportunity to make up for your cyber impression in person. It may take you a little bit longer to write a well-constructed message, but the effort will pay off. The very best leaders are always strong and precise communicators.

Lee Iacocca, one of the last quarter-century's most successful businessmen, once said, "If you want to make good use of your time, you've got to know what's important and then give it all you've got." Unfortunately, most people only follow that advice halfway. They either know what's important and then let the effort slide or they work like crazy but head in the wrong direction because they forgot to start by determining what was most important. You can choose to be different, but you must make that choice every day if you are to be truly successful.

References
1. Cooper B. The quadrant II therapist. *PT—Magazine of Physical Therapy.* 1997;5(10):30-34.
2. Covey S. *The 7 Habits of Highly Effective People.* New York, NY: Simon & Schuster; 1989.

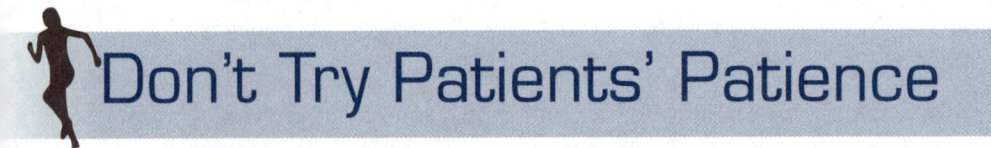

Don't Try Patients' Patience

Frustration needn't come to those who wait. Applying these principles will enhance patients' and clients' satisfaction with their visits.

In today's world of packed schedules, one thing is certain—nobody likes to wait. This is particularly true of our patients and clients. Given the fact that they're often coming to see us two or more times a week, any ill effects from making them wait are only going to multiply.

Not all forms of waiting are created equal, however. Consider the following "principles of waiting," as outlined in the book *Operations Management for MBAs*[1] and brought to my attention by a respected peer, Jon Rhodes, PT, MBA. Jon shared with me his thoughts on how these principles apply to the physical therapy clinic, and I've further tweaked them. Heeding these tips will help enhance the patient's or client's view of your practice or department, and perhaps of the entire profession. (That's another reminder that there are professional implications, direct or indirect, in most everything we do on the job.)

The principles of waiting are:

1. Unoccupied time feels longer than occupied time. What are your patients and clients doing while they're waiting? Reading a magazine? Watching a video? Sitting quietly with nothing to do? Giving them an activity that facilitates the service to come—such as asking them to complete their medical history—not only makes any wait seem shorter, but uses that time to the patient's or client's benefit.

2. Pre-service waiting feels longer than in-service waiting. Related to the first principle, this means that it's important to get the patient or client started as soon as possible in an activity related to the appointment itself. If the client is new, is there a way to get him back to the treatment room right away, where he can clothe himself accordingly and wait for the physical therapist (PT)? If this is not the patient's first visit, is there something she can start doing to prepare for therapy, such as practicing her home exercises one more time on a plinth you've made available? Can she warm up on a treadmill or UBE (upper body ergometer)?

3. Anxiety makes waiting seem longer. New clients, in particular, may be anxious not only about their dysfunction, but also about the physical therapy itself. You can help reassure them by:

- Keeping welcome packets in the waiting area that contain a letter of introduction to the clinic and short biographies of the staff, with pictures included. Instruct the receptionist to show the client the photo of the PT he or she will be seeing.

- Providing copies of APTA materials that educate patients and clients about physical therapy. Supply take-home, consumer-oriented publications such as APTA's annual consumer magazine *For Your Health* and consumer awareness brochures on preventing back and knee pain, arthritis relief, physical therapy and fitness, and other pertinent subjects. (Information on all APTA products is available at www.apta.org. Multiple copies of *For Your Health* are free to APTA members.)

- Simply dropping by the waiting room for 30 seconds to say hello to the patient or client and introducing yourself to new clients prior to the appointment.

4. Uncertain waiting is longer than known, finite waiting. Do your patients know how long they'll be waiting? Is there consistent communication between the receptionist and the clinic's PTs regarding scheduling anomalies? Does every staff PT understand and appreciate the value of momentarily stopping by the waiting room to tell a patient, "I'm running a little late; I'll be with you in less than 10 minutes"?

By reviewing your schedule at regular increments and then clearly communicating specific flow issues with your team (including receptionists and other non-PT staff), you may be able to avoid bottlenecks and reduce potential waiting times.

It's also wise to play it safe and slightly overestimate announced waits, because some patients and clients will be checking their watches constantly and will hold you to whatever you say. So, even if experience tells you the wait should be only 5 minutes, tell the patient or client "less than 10 minutes" to allow for possible delays.

5. Unexplained waiting is longer than explained waiting. For most patients and clients, the waiting goes down easier if they've been given a "why"—a reason for the delay. Ideally the explanation will come from the individual's PT, but the source isn't as important as the need for explanation.

6. Unfair waiting is longer than fair waiting. Do you have any walk-in patients? Is there ever a time in your clinic when a waiting client might observe another client coming in and being seen by a PT right away? If so, it's time to review your intake model. Consider, for example, having walk-in patients enter through a different part of the clinic from waiting patients.

7. Solo waiting is longer than group waiting. Now, don't take this one too far. You don't want clients to feel as if they're being singled out to wait, but neither do you want to create a "misery loves company" situation. Rather, think for a moment about how you can provide a congenial atmosphere in the waiting room. First of all, a friendly receptionist is worth his or her weight in gold. I've seen several in action who can turn a wait into a friendly exchange that passes the time quickly for patients and clients (and probably for the receptionist, too). Encourage such interaction, and praise it when you witness it. The other primary option here is an offshoot of principle 2. Is it possible to have a second waiting room within your gym or workout area? This not only offers patients and clients something constructive and entertaining to do while they wait, but it provides a communal setting in which time is likely to pass more quickly than it would in a typical waiting room.

8. The more valuable the service, the longer it is worth waiting for. If you're an investor you're likely familiar with the concept of the P/E ratio: Simply stated, it's a stock's price divided by its earnings per share. The higher the P/E ratio, the greater the expectation of earnings growth. What does this have to do with principle 8? Everything! Except that in this case the "P" stands for perception and the "E" stands for expectations. Think about it: If the client's perception of her experience at your clinic is low but her expectations were high, is she likely to return? By the same token, if her expectations were moderate but her perception of the visit is high, she's likely to sing your praises to others. The higher your clinic's P/E ratio, the greater the growth in your business you're likely to see taking place. Build a high P/E ratio on the first visit, and the client probably won't mind a slight wait on a subsequent visit. But create a low "client P/E" and any future wait may seem too long.

Is it time for a little "wait loss" at your facility? Take a few moments to review how the principles of waiting apply to your clinic. Handle waiting successfully, and the chances are your patients and clients will find themselves focusing on your exceptional patient care—rather than complaining about how much time it took to get to you in the first place.

Reference
1. Meredith JR, Shafer SM. *Operations Management for MBAs*. 2nd ed. Hoboken, NJ: John Wiley & Sons; 2001.

Are You Ready for a Revolution?

The days of evolutionary change in the profession are over. Prepare yourself for the ride ahead.

The next several years promise to see major changes in our profession. Trends in the economy and in health care are likely to kick-start physical therapy from gradual, evolutionary change to fast-paced, revolutionary change—change that may shake up some of our long-held beliefs about the "best" way to provide care.

Are you ready for a revolution? Let's look at a few of the changes we soon may be facing as a profession and as individual physical therapists (PTs).

Real Money

Right now, we don't deal much with "real money." Oh sure, we charge for our services, review income statements, and so on. But in most cases the payment doesn't come directly from the consumer. The patient or client essentially is spending someone else's money—the insurance company's. And, as anyone with teenagers knows, it's much easier to spend someone else's money than it is to spend one's own.

This situation is about to change drastically, however. If you haven't noticed yet, you'll soon begin to see significant increases in per-visit co-pays (from $5 to $25 or even $50) and a shift from capped co-pays to co-insurance, with the patient paying a percentage of the total per-visit cost. Also, medical savings accounts—IRA-like tax-sheltered savings plans that are lower-cost but feature higher deductibles—are appealing to more and more health care consumers and their employers.

So what, you say? So, everything! What all of this means is that there is more pressure than ever before to provide exceptional value to each and every patient or client who walks through your door. When the out-of-pocket cost of your service is only a $10 co-pay, some patients may put up with a rushed treatment session or a fill-in PT who isn't quite up to speed on that patient's particulars. At $50 out-of-pocket, however, consumer patience wears considerably thinner. If you're not providing outstanding value to the patient or client for that $50, you may not get another chance to serve him or her.

But don't see this as a negative. It effectively increases the value of truly exceptional PTs and marginalizes those who are just getting by. If you are successful in attracting and retaining patients and clients who are paying more of their costs out of pocket, your "accounts receivables" shrink because you're immediately collecting a higher percentage of the per-visit cost. And you're coming closer, in a sense, to having a single customer, rather than walking the fence between whether your "real" customer is the patient or his or her insurance company.

In this scenario, gaining approvals from insurance companies for physical therapy becomes easier, not harder. That's because insurance companies employ extensive charts that tell them how many visits the typical patient is likely to pay for, depending on the size of his or her portion of the payment. When there is no patient co-pay, the charts might indicate, for example, that the patient may make 40 to 50 visits or more. With a $5 co-pay, meanwhile, he may pursue and attend physical therapy sessions 25 times or more. At a $10 co-pay, the PT probably is looking at 12 to 18 patient visits on average. When visits hit the $50-out-of-pocket-per-visit level, the majority of patients may drop down to five to seven visits or less if they're not seeing significant improvement. Which, of course, is more to the insurance company's liking.

Along these same lines, self-pay programs will grow in importance. More and more patients will decide to go without insurance or will go the medical savings account route, both of which involve up-front out-of-pocket payments. (In fact, if you have not already implemented a reasonable self-pay program in your organization, now's the time to get started.)

So, what does this trend toward "real money" mean in relation to your practice or facility?

- If patients aren't perceiving improvement in their condition, you won't be perceiving as many visits to your clinic.

- Highly skilled therapists who are dedicated to keeping up-to-date and expanding their knowledge will be able to write their own tickets.

- Marginal therapists who merely maintain the status quo will see their value go down over time. (Fifteen years of experience will mean little, by itself, to consumers).

- Collections (net revenue) per patient will decrease, but you'll see the money faster and the authorization process will be simpler.

- You will need to demonstrate directly to the patient or client the value of your services. You'd better set what patients consider to be reasonable rates.

- Customer surveys will become more important, and the questions asked will change. "Did you have a pleasant experience?" will be supplanted by "Please rate the value of today's appointment."

Better, Not Bigger

Large therapy organizations and hospitals will continue to succeed, but they likely will look very different. Size no longer will be a natural advantage, and multiple layers of management will disappear as PTs on the front lines of patient care better understand the business side of physical therapy and feel they have a stake in the clinic's success.

As a result, managers will become teachers, not "administrators." Senior vice presidents will become "senior information sharers and trainers." They will succeed by giving power, benefits, and responsibility to those on the front lines. Organizations will become flatter, with individual PTs becoming responsible for more and more aspects of their clinic. With that responsibility, however, also will come opportunities for PTs to shape their futures and their clinics' direction.

Because organizations will be flatter and less hierarchical, PTs will remain in clinical positions for much longer periods rather than moving out of clinical care into management. It will be increasingly important, therefore, for organizations to take full advantage of PTs' skill, knowledge, and maturity by developing and expanding mentoring programs and internal development opportunities.

You're in Charge of Your Career

For far too long, PTs have depended on natural progression to grow professionally. As the company grew, their responsibilities did, too. As they gained years of experience, their salaries increased accordingly.

No more. Now it's up to you. Your years of experience mean less than what you've actually learned, the ways in which you've stretched yourself, and how you've really grown. Otherwise, you may not be anything more, professionally, than an "old new grad."

Let it rain! If you're a rainmaker who can bring in patients, you'll also bring home a higher salary. If you are not building relationships with referral sources and getting your expertise known in your area, then your professional options are likely to be stunted. But if you are successfully building those relationships, the sky's the limit.

Organizational chart? What organizational chart? Titles will become less meaningful. The most influential people in your company, regardless of its size, will be those who are well thought-of and have the fullest Rolodexes. Do referral sources and peers call you for assistance? What do people in your organization who have never spent time with you think of you? What are you doing each day to expand your network? Ask yourself:

- Do you really have 15 years of experience, or is it 1 year of experience repeated 15 times?

- How many physicians refer to your facility because of you? How could you triple that number?

- How large is your "impact circle?" Does your reputation and influence spread beyond the patients you treat to the surrounding community?

- What have you done this past year to stretch your skills, talent, and knowledge?

- What are you known for as a PT? Your manual skills? Your entrepreneurial expertise? Your strong referral relationships with physicians? Your advocacy for the profession through APTA?

- What will you be known for a year from now? (Something new?)

- Do you understand how your company works? Can you read an income statement? What key indicators drive the success or failure of your facility? If you're going to be assuming more responsibility for that success or failure, you'd better understand the basics.

The Web Rules

Do you think the computer revolution ended with the dot-com crash? Think again. The Internet is hot, and will continue to be! If we don't recognize that, we'll be passed by as a profession.

Patients are coming into our clinics far better educated than ever before. They're going online and looking up everything from their own medical condition to the skinny on the physical therapy facility. If you don't have a presence on the Web, that would be a good item to put near the top of your priority list. And by a "presence" I'm not talking about a simple home page with your name and telephone number. I'm talking about:

- Biographies of all of your facility's PTs and PTAs.
- Online scheduling capability.
- A package available for purchase at discharge that allows the patient to e-mail questions to his or her PT and schedule a screening within 24 hours.
- Patient and client accessibility—from home, work, and perhaps a Web-enabled kiosk in your waiting room—to the following conveniences and information: automated check-in and co-pay payment via credit card; confirmation of the number of approved visits; a spot to enter the date of the physician follow-up visit; the ability to order any supplies, to be shipped to the patient's home the same day; self-scheduling services; the ability to access a diagnosis and print or e-mail that information to the patient's own e-mail address; and the means to provide completely anonymous (and immediate!) feedback on services provided.

A Shift in Quadrants

The story of the Saturn automobile has gotten a great deal of attention over the years, but it's worth revisiting as we look at our own industry. General Motors, one of the largest car companies in the world (did you even know that the cute little Saturn was part of a huge corporation?) took a close look at its products and realized it had plenty of cars that were:

- Conservative in style and economical in price.
- Conservative in style and expensive in price.
- Sporty in style and expensive in price.

What was missing? GM realized it had neglected an entire quadrant of the market: sporty in style and economical in price. Oops! So it began work on what was to become Saturn. There are many reasons the new make succeeded, but one of the most important ones is the fact that GM addressed its primary gap.

How about us? PTs' quadrants are a bit different, but four distinct areas nevertheless emerge:

- The patient's payment is covered by insurance and he or she receives passive treatment by the PT.

- The patient's payment is covered by insurance and he or she receives active treatment by the PT.

- The patient pays out-of-pocket and receives passive treatment by the PT.

- The patient pays out-of-pocket and receives active treatment by the PT.

Treatment Given by a PT And How it is Paid for

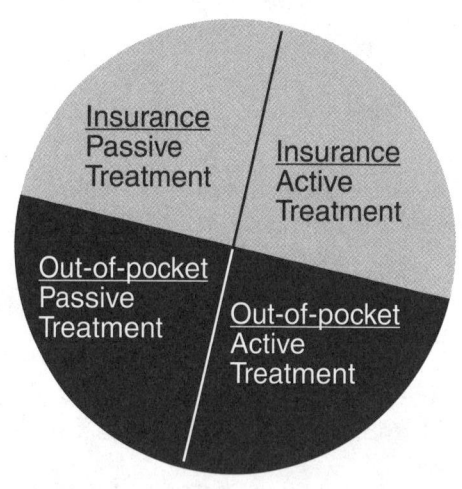

(Pie chart with quadrants: Insurance Passive Treatment, Insurance Active Treatment, Out-of-pocket Passive Treatment, Out-of-pocket Active Treatment)

I'm convinced that, for the most part, we've ignored not merely one quadrant but half the market: self-payers! We took the easy way of the third-party payer. And now many of us are about to face the shredder. Not the revolutionaries among us, however. They saw this opportunity and sacrificed time, energy, and maybe even some money on the third-party payer side, but now they're ahead of the curve. They're well positioned for the future. Can you say the same?

Some Things Are Timeless

Not everything will change. There are at least three aspects of your work as a PT that always will benefit you, through evolutionary and revolutionary times alike: clinical expertise, solid relationships with patients and clients, and maintenance of a strong personal network of contacts. If you have all three you'll likely be successful through every bump and twist along the way.

I don't have a crystal ball, but one thing is for certain. If we are to survive and thrive, we cannot continue doing things the way we've always done them. The future promises to be a bit of a wild ride, but it'll be a lot easier to navigate if you've got your hands on the steering wheel.

What's for Lunch? How About Innovation?

Maybe you can't "shrink your way to greatness," but you can put it on your menu.

"You can't shrink your way to greatness!" shouted Tom Peters from the jacket of *The Circle of Innovation*.[1] That book was published in 1997, when cost-cutting was everything, but Peters warned that creativity was needed to take advantage of the resulting opportunities.

But even in better economic times for physical therapy and other professions and businesses, the need for new approaches is every bit as critical. And that starts with your day-to-day actions.

The time for greatness is now! But it won't come if you always follow the pack. Now is the time for true innovators to move to the front, to stand out from the crowd, to champion their cause, their skills, and their profession.

The perplexing thing about innovation is that while we know on an abstract level that it's vital to the long-term success of any organization, on a personal level we often are hesitant to exercise it. But innovative vision requires a new outlook, a new mindset, a commitment to go beyond the ordinary, a willingness to break free of the curve and shout, "I refuse to fit into that box!"

Do you think you're ready to pursue innovation? Let's find out. What are your answers to the following questions?

- Do you always drive the same way to work?
- Do you tend to eat lunch at the same place, with the same people?
- What did you have for lunch today, anyway? Did it by any chance resemble what you had yesterday and the day before?
- What are your plans for the upcoming weekend? Are you experiencing déjà vu just thinking about them?

The point is, greatness requires a change in habits. Michael Jordan didn't simply wake up one morning and say, "You know what? I think I'll become the greatest basketball player in the history of the game" and have it come to fruition. Rather, while he certainly was blessed with amazing natural talent, he also chose to do things differently—from his personal training program and diet to his high-intensity workouts on the court. Only then did his dream become a reality.

> Your new route to work might reveal a billboard you'd never seen, which in turn might remind you of a program idea you'd considered but hadn't pursued.

So, change a habit or two, just for experimentation's sake. Break out of your everyday patterns, and innovation may blossom. Your new route to work might reveal a billboard you'd never seen, which in turn might remind you of a program idea you'd considered but hadn't pursued. The new employee you invite to lunch might know someone whose ideas nicely supplement your own. The new dish you try and later rave about to co-workers might draw into conversation a co-worker with whom you hadn't spoken before—your future collaborator, perhaps. And your weekend drive up into the mountains with the windows down may inspire your creativity in ways that another afternoon spent in front of the TV never would have. I think you'll be very pleasantly surprised by the results of any or all such small modifications of your routine, even if you just diverge from your norm on an occasional basis.

Another early step to innovation is to step back, in a sense. A good friend of mine once passed along the sage advice that success as a manager requires working *on* your business, not necessarily always *in* your business. The point is, when you're completely immersed in the daily aspects of running a practice or facility, it may be difficult to raise your nose from the grindstone long enough to look around and identify things that need changing.

One effective way to approach change-making is to ... blow it up! No, I'm not talking about detonating your building in hopes of collecting the insurance money! Rather, I'm encouraging you to mentally step outside of your organization and let the status quo disappear from your mind's eye. Then start over. Rebuild from the ground up, with new materials that include innovative programs, ideas, and services. Ask yourself what you would do differently were you starting from scratch. Consider which programs you'd revive if only you could. (Because, guess what? Chances are you can.)

Most important, identify innovative programs you could bring to life with the resources now available to you, to supplement or enhance your current offerings. And think about what you need to do to get those programs started. (If you can't identify any innovative programs, maybe it's time to change your commute again, or try some new dishes at lunchtime!)

It's been said that a fool is someone who does the same things over and over but expects different results each time. Innovators try different things—new things, unexpected things—every day. They know that life holds no guarantees, except that those who remain in their ruts never will achieve the greatness that lies above and beyond them.

Reference

1. Peters T. *The Circle of Innovation*. New York, NY: Vintage Books; 1997.

Up-to-the-Minute Advice

You can't make time stand still, but you can use it to better advantage without making major changes in your schedule.

Feeling busy? No time to spare? Find yourself racing from Monday morning to Friday night with little time to take a breath? Have your New Year's resolutions regarding personal fitness, relationships, spiritual pursuits, or/and advanced education already fallen by the wayside—victims of the "busy-ness of your business" as a physical therapist (PT) or physical therapist assistant (PTA)?

You're not alone. Life's demanding—packed with activities, pressures, and obligations from all sides. But I've learned that there are plenty of things anyone can start doing today to free up time that instead can be devoted to your top priorities in life.

Not that I've got it all figured out. Please! My time's spread awfully thin. I'm a husband and the father of three growing kids, my job keeps me busy 50-60 hours a week, I write books and speak about leadership all over the country, I train for and compete in triathlons, and I'm deeply involved in my local church. Sometimes I hit the wall and stumble. But precisely because my life's so frenetic, I've come up with some time-stretching strategies that may help you, too.

- *Envisioning.* Do you have a vision—a clear picture in your mind's eye of how you want your life to look? The way to sculpt a work of art is to visualize the end result and chip away all the extra stone. So, too, must you clear away impediments to your ideal future as someone who has the time to accomplish not only everything that must be done, but also all those things you most want to do.

- *Sleeping.* Think about going to bed earlier, even if by just a half-hour. When I tell people that I get up at 4:30 am in order to hit the pool before work, most of them look at me like I have two heads! But the key isn't what time you get up, it's what time you turn in. Getting up at 4:30 am is easy (well, maybe not "easy," but not too hard) if you're in bed by 9:30 pm.

    Most people spend their last couple of waking hours each day sitting in front of the television set. So, if there's a pursuit you'd like to add to your life that could take place first thing in the morning—such as exercise, for instance, recognizing that we are *physical* therapists and *physical* therapist assistants—consider a tradeoff with the TV. You can record the shows you miss and watch them later, anyway! Also, you can trim 20 minutes from

Section 6 — Greet the Clock

every hour you spend in front of the TV by using available technology to skip the commercials. Those time savings may facilitate your turning in earlier—and thus arising earlier, too.

- **Driving.** What about your commuting time? It takes me 35 minutes to drive to the office in rush-hour traffic. But getting up at 4:30, I head into town well before rush hour, and the trip takes me less than 15 minutes. I'm not saying you can or should start seeing patients at 5 am. (You probably wouldn't get many takers!) But, could you shift your starting time even slightly, save some minutes on the road as a result, and use that time more profitably? It's something to consider. If you have access to a shower at work, perhaps you could you arrive early and work out at the office. Or, maybe a gym or health club near your clinic could serve the same purpose. Perhaps, instead, you could do some early-morning grocery shopping, putting items that must be kept cold in your refrigerator at work. If you have more than a few such items, maybe you even could leave them in the supermarket's cooler. I worked for a grocery store when I was in high school, and we were happy to let good customers store items for the day.

How about meeting a friend for breakfast downtown, or spending some early-morning quiet time solo at a restaurant or in your office chair, catching up on all those back issues of *PT—Magazine of Physical Therapy* you've been saving for "someday?" Get creative—but get out of traffic. Often a mere 30-minute shift in starting time can have a huge impact on the amount of time you must spend in the car.

Speaking of time spent on the road, why not make it productive? Have you been wanting to catch up on books you've been hearing about? Why not pick them up on CD, or download them to your iPod? I just picked up the CD of the bestseller *The Purpose-Driven Life*[1] and have been listening to it on my way to the pool before work. Maybe I'm only in the car for 15 minutes, but it has become a purpose-driven quarter-hour!

One more "car suggestion." Obesity is a huge problem in this country—one we're facing more and more in our profession. Among the many factors contributing to overweight are tight schedules that force people on the run to grab the first thing available. If you don't have time to eat a good breakfast at home, keep a few bags of almonds, raisins, or healthy trail mix in your car to eat during your morning commute. Keeping nutritional foods in the car also may reduce the temptation to duck into a fast-food place for lunch if you're out running errands at midday. You should see the floor of my car—it looks like a miniature health food store!

- ***Planning.*** Dedicate time on your schedule to the things that are most important to you, professionally and personally. If you allot time to those priorities long before your day planner is completely packed, they can't as easily be crowded out of your itinerary. And once you establish certain priorities as "givens" on your calendar, you'll likely be amazed at how smoothly lesser (but still important) parts of your daily itinerary will fall into place around those "must-dos." Practice makes perfect. It used to take me 15 minutes each night to pack my workout gear and business attire for the following morning. Now I put everything I'll need for the week in a bag that I draw from each workday. Look at the things you do regularly and focus on making those activities more efficient.
- ***Pack a lunch.*** Not only will the dollars saved add up, but so will the time saved. And chances are you'll find yourself eating a healthier meal than you would have had you gone out. How's that for a triple-threat benefit?

Join in! You're treating patients most of the day, so why not treat yourself in the process? Most patients love it when PTs and PTAs get involved to the point of doing some of the exercises along with them, and you'll be enhancing your own health in the process. Also, if you sit at a desk much of the day, substitute a Swiss ball for your chair for a few hours. You'll be enhancing your core stability without spending any extra time exercising.

Take care of yourself. If you drove a racecar, you wouldn't fill it with junk fuel or load it down with luggage, would you? Well, you're essentially running a race each and every day. If you fill yourself with good fuel, shed extra pounds, and keep an eye on your overall maintenance, you'll have more energy and a sharper focus for meeting the demands of each and every day.

Face it, life's not going to slow down anytime soon. But we each have it within our power to spend our time in the most fulfilling and productive ways possible. Sleep on that thought. And while you're at it, think about turning in a little earlier tonight!

References
1. Warren R. *The Purpose-Driven Life: What on Earth Am I Here For?* Grand Rapids, Mich: Zondervan Publishing Company; 2002.

Bringing It All Back Home

Ruminations on physical therapy as a bridge among past, present, and future.

Lured by a program of special alumni events, I returned recently to the city where I had attended graduate school. It had been a long time since I'd last driven down those streets, but, as I did, the memories came flooding back.

There was the hole-in-the-wall apartment I'd shared with two roommates in order to save money. It may have been a dump, but it also was home base for intriguing discussions, creative meals, some practical jokes, and even a few tears.

There was the cobblestone street on which I first broached the subject of "the future" with a girlfriend. And there was the huge park through which I biked and ran with my friends, long before I ever entered my first triathlon.

As I drove through this familiar city for the first time in years, I kept thinking of the saying "you can't go home again." I suppose the wider validity of that statement is different for every individual, but I was struck by this related thought about our profession: One of the big reasons physical therapy has become such a critical and valued part of the health care continuum is that it does, in essence, allow patients to "go home again."

Think about it. Physical therapy, for many people, is the ultimate time machine. In a very real sense, physical therapists (PTs) and physical therapist assistants (PTAs) help transport patients and clients back to the "good old days." Maybe not back to the days of their youth, but back to more-recent, happier times when they were more mobile and perhaps in some ways more alive.

Our role in "time travel" is enormous. We help bring athletes back home to their passion, whether it's running, cycling, swimming, tennis, golf, or what have you. We help bring injured workers back home to their livelihoods. We help make our patients' home lives all that they were before injury limited their activities and interactions with their loved ones.

And PTs' and PTAs' role in time travel goes well beyond the physical. The structure and encouragement we provide can help return patients—for the length of their clinic visit, anyway—to what may seem a bygone era. The country music hit "Mayberry" by Rascal Flatts fondly harks back to the days when things were gentler and daily life was a whirl of smiles and first names, rather than road rage and impersonality. Well, our profession reclaims a little bit of that world for the people we serve.

Our patients may not be able to control the stock market's fluctuations, prevent their bosses' irrational outbursts, or successfully influence all the choices their kids make, but for the time they're with us—a group of caring professionals who not only have the education, training, and skills to help them get better physically, but also the genuine interest in them and their progress to reassure them and ease their fears—they're back home, in a place that looks less like the sets of those backbiting "reality" TV shows of today and more like the Mayberry that Andy Griffith put on the airwaves 40-something years ago.

But you know, when it comes to time travel, we also serve as springboards to our patients' futures. We safeguard them against injury and give them the knowledge and tools they need to embrace new fitness pursuits, hobbies, even professional options, with reduced health risk and increased opportunity for accomplishment and enjoyment.

One final thought from my reunion weekend: Each of us tends to get a little lost or misdirected the farther from "home" we travel, whether in our personal or professional lives. What if we went back to the early days of marriage and treated our spouses the way we did when love was new? Similarly, do you remember your first week on the job as a PT or PTA? You wanted to make a difference! You wanted to make a positive impact! Is that enthusiasm still there? If not, why not? What did you do then that you don't do now? Would your younger self admire the PT or PTA you've become? Would that eager rookie you once were see room for improvement? If so, in what areas?

You get the idea. In a way, we all can go home again. In fact, it can be a very important part of moving forward. Which is something about which PTs and PTAs know an awful lot.

Suggested Reading

Ailes R. *You Are the Message.* New York, NY: Doubleday; 1995.

Beckwith H. *Selling the Invisible.* Holbrook, Mass: Bob Adams Inc; 1994.

Bennis W, Nanus B. *Leaders: Strategies for Taking Charge.* New York, NY: HarperBusiness; 1997.

Berens LV, Ernst L, Smith M. *The Guide for Facilitating the Self-Discovery Process.* Huntington Beach, Calif: Temperament Research Institute; 2000.

Berens LV, Nardi D. *The 16 Personality Types: Descriptions for Self-Discovery.* Huntington Beach, Calif: Telos Publications; 1999.

Berens LV, Ernst L, Robb J, Smith M. *Temperament and Type Dynamics: The Facilitator's Guide.* Huntington Beach, Calif: Telos Publications; 1998.

Berens, LV. *Understanding Yourself and Others: An Introduction to Temperament.* Huntington Beach, Calif: Temperament Research Institute; 1998.

Boe A. *Is Your "Net" Working?* New York, NY: John Wiley and Sons; 1989.

Buckingham M, Coffman C. *First, Break All the Rules: What the World's Greatest Managers Do Differently.* New York, NY: Simon & Schuster; 1999.

Buckingham M, Clifton DO. *Now, Discover Your Strengths.* New York, NY: Free Press; 2001.

Clason G. *The Richest Man in Babylon.* New York, NY: Bantam Books; 1989 (reissue).

Cooper B. *Quick Guide to Four Temperaments and Sales.* Hunting Beach, Calif: Telos Publications; 2003.

Cooper B, Berens LV. *Groundbreaking Sales Skills: Portable Sales Techniques to Ensure Success.* Huntington Beach, Calif: Telos Publications; 2004.

Cooper RK. *The Other 90%: How to Unlock Your Vast Untapped Potential for Leadership and Life.* New York, NY: Crown Publishing; 2001.

Covey S. *Principle-Centered Leadership.* New York, NY: Fireside; 1992.

Covey S. *The 7 Habits of Highly Effective People.* New York, NY: Simon & Schuster; 1989.

Eldredge J. *Wild at Heart: Discovering the Secret of a Man's Soul.* Nashville, Tenn: Thomas Nelson, Inc; 2001.

Fisher D, Vilas S. *Power Networking.* Austin, Texas: MountainHarbour Publications; 1991.

Frankl VE. *Man's Search for Meaning.* Boston, Mass: Beacon Press; 2000.

Gates B. *Business @ the Speed of Thought: Succeeding in the Digital Age.* New York, NY: Warner Books; 2000.

Gitomer J. *Customer Satisfaction Is Worthless, Customer Loyalty Is Priceless.* Austin, Texas: Bard Press; 1998.

Goldratt E. *The Goal.* Great Barrington, Mass: North River Press; 1984.

Harding F. *Rain Making: The Professional's Guide to Attracting New Clients.* Holbrook, Mass: Adams Media; 1994.

Harvey G. Networking Smart. Presented at: Denver Chamber of Commerce meeting; January 27, 2000; Denver, Colorado.

Keirsey D. *Please Understand Me II: Temperament, Character, Intelligence.* Del Mar, Calif: Prometheus Nemesis Book Co; 1998.

Keirsey D, Bates M. *Please Understand Me.* Del Mar, Calif: Prometheus Nemesis Book Company; 1978.

Krannich CR, Krannich RL. *Dynamite Networking for Dynamite Jobs.* Manassas Park, Va: Impact Publications; 1996.

Leboeuf M. *How to Win Customers and Keep Them for Life [audiotape].* New York, NY: Simon and Schuster; 1997.

Lencioni PM. *The Four Obsessions of an Extraordinary Executive.* San Francisco, Calif: Jossey-Bass; 2000.

MacKay H. *Dig Your Well Before You're Thirsty.* New York, NY: Doubleday; 1997.

Meredith JR, Shafer SM. *Operations Management for MBAs.* 2nd ed. Hoboken, NJ: John Wiley & Sons; 2001.

Peters T. *The Brand You 50.* New York, NY: Random House; 1999.

Peters T. *The Circle of Innovation.* New York, NY: Vintage Books; 1999.

Roane S. *How to Work a Room.* New York, NY: Audio Renaissance; 1991.

Vilas S, Fisher D. *Power Networking: 55 Secrets for Personal and Professional Success.* Austin, Texas: Bard Press; 1992.

Warren R. *The Purpose-Driven Life: What on Earth Am I Here For?* Grand Rapids, Mich: Zondervan Publishing Company; 2002.

Weil A. *Eating Well for Optimum Health.* New York, NY: Alfred A Knopf; 2000.

Ziglar Z. *Top Performance: How to Develop Excellence in Yourself and Others.* New York, NY: Berkley Publishing Group; 1991.

SOUTH UNIVERSITY - RICHMOND

35019002210473